MARATHON

MARATHON
The Ultimate Training and Racing Guide

By Hal Higdon,
Senior Writer, *Runner's World* Magazine

Rodale Press, Emmaus, Pennsylvania

OUR MISSION

We publish books that empower people's lives.

RODALE 🌱 BOOKS

"High-Carbohydrate Foods" on pages 114–15 was adapted from *Nancy Clark's Sports Nutrition Guidebook,* by Nancy Clark, with permission from the author.

"Oxygen Power Table" on pages 126–27 was adapted from *Oxygen Power,* by Jack Tupper Daniels and Jimmy Rhett Gilbert, with permission from the authors.

"Myers Performance Prediction Table" on page 129 and "Myers Pace Table for 3:00 Marathon" on page 134 were reprinted with permission from the author.

Cover design: Stan Green
Cover photo: Rich Cruse
Book design: Ayers/Johanek, Publication Design

If you have any questions or comments concerning this book, please write:
Rodale Press
Book Readers' Service
33 East Minor St.
Emmaus, PA 18098

Library of Congress Cataloging-in-Publication Data

Higdon, Hal.
 Marathon : the ultimate training and racing guide / by Hal Higdon.
  p. cm.
 Includes index.
 ISBN 0-87596-159-2 paperback
 1. Marathon running. 2. Marathon running–Training. I. Title.
 GB1065.H54 1993
 796.42'5–dc20   92-41569
                                                      CIP

Distributed in the book trade by St. Martin's Press

     10   paperback

In memory of
the Self-Made Olympian:
Ron Daws

CONTENTS

ACKNOWLEDGMENTS

The following coaches contributed information based on their experience as runners and with runners. The author thanks each and every one.

Dan Ashimine (Gardena, California)
Wayne E. Baldwin, Jr. (Kirkwood, Missouri)
Roy Benson (Atlanta, Georgia)
Jay Birmingham (Alamosa, Colorado)
Mark S. Bredenbaugh (West Columbia, South Carolina)
Clark Campbell (Lawrence, Kansas)
Joe Catalano (East Walpole, Massachusetts)
Mike Caton (El Paso, Texas)
Happy Chapman (Honolulu, Hawaii)
David Cowein (Morrilton, Arkansas)
Daniel Deyo (Saline, Mississippi)
Greg A. Domantay (Lake Forest, Illinois)
Sue Ellis (Holland, Michigan)
Robert Eslick (Nashville, Tennessee)
Lee Fidler (Stone Mountain, Georgia)
Dan French (Iowa City, Iowa)
Joe Friel (Fort Collins, Colorado)
Jeff Galloway (Atlanta, Georgia)
John Joseph Garvey (Oklahoma City, Oklahoma)
Ted Giampietro (Bitburg, Germany)
Paul Goss (Foster City, California)
Tom Grogon (Cincinnati, Ohio)
Nobuya Hashizume (Minnetonka, Minnesota)
Fritz Ingram (Roseburg, Oregon)
Brad Jaeger (Baltimore, Maryland)

Teri Jordan (State College, Pennsylvania)
Susan Kinsey (La Mesa, California)
Henry Laskau (Coconut Creek, Florida)
Steve Linsenbardt (Springfield, Missouri)
Frank X. Mari (Toms River, New Jersey)
Ken Martin (Sante Fe, New Mexico)
Ben Adams Moore, Jr. (Annapolis, Maryland)
Alfred F. Morris (Washington, D.C.)
Tim Nicholls (Pembroke Pines, Florida)
Gary O'Daniels (Creston, Iowa)
Diane Palmason (Englewood, Colorado)
Danny Perez (Norwalk, California)
Gaylord E. Quigley (St. Louis, Missouri)
James Redfield (Salt Lake City, Utah)
Doug Renner (Westminster, Maryland)
Dennis J. D. Robinson (Dayton, Ohio)
Craig B. Sanders (Simi Valley, California)
Rich Sands (Longmont, Colorado)
Patrick Joseph Savage (Oak Park, Illinois)
Will Shaw (Beverly, West Virginia)
Daryl J. Smith (Newburgh, New York)
Sherwin Sosnovsky (Pomona, California)
Jim Spivey (Glen Ellyn, Illinois)
Roy Stevenson (Bothell, Washington)
Drew Sutcliffe (Eugene, Oregon)
Laszlo Tabori (Culver City, California)
Judy Tillapaugh (Fort Wayne, Indiana)
John E. Tolbert (New Haven, Connecticut)
Gary Tuttle (Dover, New Hampshire)
Joy Upshaw-Margerum (Kamuela, Hawaii)
Robert H. Vaughan (Dallas, Texas)
David W. Virtue (Westwood Hills, Kansas)
Robert Wallace (Dallas, Texas)
William Wenmark (Deephaven, Minnesota)
Danny White (Marion, South Carolina)
Bob Williams (Portland, Oregon)
Keith Woodard (Portland, Oregon)
Richard Wotawa (Berkshire, New York)

INTRODUCTION

At the awards ceremony after a race in South Bend, Indiana, I chatted with Mary Connolly, one of northwestern Indiana's top runners. She praised an article by me in that month's *Runner's World* titled "The Road to Recovery" that described how to bounce back more quickly after a marathon.

"I wish you had written that article ten years ago," Mary chided me. "It took me that long to learn what you wrote."

I smiled: "It took me *30* years."

So true. In April 1959, I arrived in Boston to run my first race of 26 miles and 385 yards. I knew nothing about pace, so I just tried to keep up with the fast Finnish and Japanese runners I saw at the starting line. I walked off the course at 18 miles. That was my first experience at hitting the "Wall."

Better training would do the trick, I reasoned. Except back in the Dark Ages of road racing in the United States, few people knew much about "better training." Most coaches knew only track techniques. There were no classes for first-time marathoners. There were no books dispensing advice. Who would read them? The Road Runners Club of America consisted of a half dozen of us meeting in a tiny hotel room in New York the afternoon of the indoor track championships. I experimented with high mileage and many interval quarters run on the track. I didn't finish my next two marathon attempts—Culver City, California, and Boston—and got to the finish line of marathon number four in Yonkers, New York, only because no drivers would stop for me when I tried to hitchhike at mile 24.

Now you're probably thinking: With a record like that, he's going to try to teach *me* how to run the marathon?

Well, eventually I *did* learn how to run this event. Through trial and error, I discovered how to train properly and returned to Boston in 1964 to finish fifth—the first American—with a time of 2:21:55 that remains my personal record. But I still didn't understand proper diet: One diary entry from that era shows that I ate steak as a prerace meal! It seems ludicrous now, but the prerace pasta feast had not yet become a part of the long-distance runner's ritual.

In 1968 I participated with several other runners in what would be recognized later as *the* landmark fluid replacement study for marathoners, an ongoing study that culminated at the Olympic Marathon trials in Alamosa, Colorado. The study was conducted by David L. Costill, Ph.D., director of the then-unsung Human Performance Laboratory at Ball State University in Muncie, Indiana. Dr. Costill wanted to provide us with fluids every 5 kilometers in the race. Knowledgeable marathoners today might ask: Why wait until 5 kilometers? But international regulations back then prohibited runners even from taking any water before *15* kilometers!

Unfortunately, race officials reneged on an agreement and informed Dr. Costill only after we were off and running that he could not give liquids before the 15-K mark. To do so would result in our disqualification, something Dr. Costill hardly wanted to risk. At 5 kilometers, I reached for water and discovered Dave standing with empty hand and an embarrassed expression. Dehydrated and well behind the leaders, I dropped out again. The results of Dr. Costill's research, however, eventually prompted changes in the international rules to permit the frequent refreshment stations that today's runners take for granted.

Much of my running career preceded the knowledge that today makes marathon running accessible to the masses as well as the elite. During my embryonic years as a long-distance runner, no mass-circulation magazines existed to dispense advice to runners or, for that matter, athletes in any fitness sport. It was not until 1966 that *Distance Running News* (later renamed *Runner's World*) appeared, starting as a newsletter and taking a dozen years to achieve prominence among the growing running community. Only then could a Mary Connolly open an issue and learn during a few minutes of reading what it had taken many pioneer runners—drawing on the advice of coaches, scientists and other runners—years or even decades to learn.

My coming of age as a marathoner occurred January 14, 1981, at the World Veterans Championships in Christchurch, New Zealand. After a series of successes and failures over the previous quarter century, I had become a competent and confident marathoner. I had aged, my legs had lost some of their youthful snap, but I could compensate somewhat with improved knowledge.

I had come to the starting line following 18 months of careful preparation, ready to run well that particular day. I had done my long runs. I had done my speedwork. I had rested when necessary. I knew about pace. I had mastered the necessary arts of nutrition and fluid replacement. I was ready.

On a warm and breezy day, I let my rivals in the 45-to-49 age group move away from me early on. I shepherded my energies. At each aid station, I walked while drinking to make sure I got enough fluid. As the race progressed, I kept aware of how I felt and how far away my age-group rivals were. I waited. Midway through the race, I began to pass runners: It was not so much that I sped up as that they slowed down. I crossed the finish line tenth overall and won my age group by nearly three minutes. I was the world champion. My time of 2:29:27 at age 49 actually was the second fastest during my career and represented a triumph of accumulated knowledge, rather than merely talent. And similar triumphs are available to every reader of this book, since most of us measure ourselves not against a few fast marathoners but against our own abilities.

Although many runners limit their marathon forays to once or twice a year, rather than the five or six they might have run at the peak of the running boom a decade ago, the marathon is still popular. In 1990, according to Basil and Linda Honikman of TACSTATS, the 10-K was the most popular race distance, with 1,208,000 finishers. The marathon ranked fourth, with 263,000 reported finishers—a solid base of support (5-K and 8-K were second and third). There are now 521 certified marathon courses in the United States, with about 50 new ones certified each year. In terms of prize money, the marathon is kingpin of the professional circuit, awarding nearly two-thirds of the prize money ($3,938,000 of $6,065,206 in 1991).

I continue to run at least one or two marathons a year—although I don't necessarily always try to run them hard or achieve a top performance. I simply love marathons. I enjoy the experience, the camaraderie that transcends that found in shorter races. Perhaps the greatest benefit of running marathons is the focus it gives to your training. It forces you to do the things—such as long Sunday runs—that you probably want to do anyway.

But you don't have to run marathons to run far. One of my favorite distances is the 15-K, the distance of the Michigan City Run that I founded in 1965. It is the oldest road race in Indiana and just happens to run by my front door.

I also enjoy half-marathons, which provide much of the pleasure and less of the pain of full marathons. Among my favorite runs are two 25-K races: the popular Old Kent River Bank Run in Grand Rapids, Michigan, in May and a lesser-known race along the banks of the Illinois and Michigan Canal in Channahon, Illinois, in September. One of the National AAU Championships I won was the 30-K, in 1964 in Silver Springs, Maryland, and the national 30-K record I later set for the 40-to-44 age group lasted 16 years. I've raced only occasionally past the marathon distance in ultramarathons, but wish I had more time to explore longer roads and trails.

Marathon comes on the heels—and serves as an extension—of *Run Fast,* my 1992 performance guide for running distances of ten kilometers and less. Just as *Run Fast* guided those seeking speed and glory over short road distances, *Marathon* will do the same for those who want to move on to longer distances, particularly the marathon. This book will let you maximize your potential in running 26 miles and 385 yards.

In researching this book, I have had the help of approximately 60 of the most knowledgeable coaches in America, who coach runners of all ages and abilities. Several years ago I wrote an article in *Runner's World* called "The Coach Approach," suggesting that most runners could benefit from the help of a coach. After the article appeared, we collected the names of coaches all over the United States. Executive editor Amby Burfoot considers this group a rich source of wisdom on the art of running.

For this book I tapped into this source, and more than 50

coaches responded with completed questionnaires. Among the respondents:

- Joe Catalano of East Walpole, Massachusetts, who has coached world-class runners, including his former wife, Patti Lyons Catalano, a 2:27:50 marathoner.
- Jeff Galloway, a coach of first-time runners and a former Olympian.
- Teri Jordan, the head track and cross-country coach at Pennsylvania State University, the fourth-ranked marathoner in the world in 1973.
- Ken Martin of Santa Fe, New Mexico, a 2:09:38 marathoner.

Many other experienced coaches whose names are not well known also responded. For the most part, these are not high school or college track coaches but are among a growing number of individuals who work with out-of-school runners of both exceptional and ordinary talents.

Not all of their responses could be easily summarized statistically, but you will encounter the wisdom of these respondents throughout the remainder of this book, and I have made much use of their expertise.

This book is also a compilation of all I have learned, not only from my racing but from the experts of the runner's world. The knowledge I found so difficult (and painful) to acquire in years past now is available to those who want to test their talents at this classic distance. I hope *Marathon* permits you more enjoyment (and better times) the next time you, too, run far.

CHAPTER 1

The Mystique of the
MARATHON

I heard the comment in passing, approximately eight miles into the Twin Cities Marathon. "To think," said a woman spectator, "they paid to do this." Her comment floated out of the crowd, but by the time I turned to look, my stride had carried me past where she stood beside the course.

I understood what she meant. Twenty-six miles *is* a long way. Even thinking about running that far takes a certain amount of endurance. Yet somehow those of us who call ourselves marathoners do it again, and again, and again.

The woman's comment at Twin Cities about paying to destroy our bodies didn't disturb me. First of all, I thought there was some truth to it. Second, I was too busy running as fast as I could to worry about what spectators thought.

Only later would her remark return to haunt me. It was obvious that she failed to comprehend the mystique of the marathon. Yet how do you fully explain to spectators the joy and pain that goes into running the marathon distance of 26 miles and 385 yards?

The woman certainly would have found ludicrous the personal quest on which I had just embarked. As a 60th birthday challenge, I had decided to run six marathons on six successive weekends. Twin Cities—in Minneapolis—was merely the first of the six. The effort almost destroyed me, and I came close to dropping out of several of the races. Reporters asked if my six-in-six stunt was a world record for successive marathons. I smiled, because obviously they had never heard of Sy Mah, who in his lifetime finished 524 marathons. (More about him later.)

Sy Mah would have understood my obsession with running marathons. He knew that it's not merely the race itself but also the preparation that goes into the race: the steady buildup of miles, the long runs on Sundays, the inevitable taper, the ceremonial aspects of the total experience. One positive aspect of marathoning is that it provides focus for your training and offers a recognizable goal.

The woman watching us race at Twin Cities probably would shake her head in disbelief if told by any of the 5,076 finishers that day that they had enjoyed the experience, that it had been fun. *Fun* isn't a word that occurs to most nonmarathoners when they consider the marathon.

Doug Kurtis understands, however. Kurtis, 40, lives in Northville, Michigan; he is a systems analyst for the Ford Motor Company. As of October 1992, he had run 131 marathons, finishing 66 faster than 2:20. In a typical year, he runs a dozen marathons. One year at the Barcelona Marathon, he went out too hard on a hot day and faded to eighth. The Danish race winner asked him afterward, "Was that one fun?"

Kurtis had to admit that it wasn't, but he said he wouldn't run a dozen marathons a year if he didn't think they were fun. "Often, the enjoyment is the training before and the memory after," he says.

Like Kurtis, I believe the actual running of the marathon is secondary to the training leading up to the event. If you love to run, then you appreciate the motivation the marathon provides for those long Sunday runs and those fast midweek track workouts. Marathon training focuses the mind, and that may be the best excuse for racing this distance.

"I go out for my daily workouts because I enjoy running," says Kurtis. "At noon, I pick scenic routes through surrounding streets near my office. In the evening, I often run from home along a parkway. I like to find pleasant places to run and see the sights. I enjoy being out there day after day. Races are just a by-product."

Marathon Immunity

Marathon running also has the potential to increase life span and to increase the quality of that life span. Again, it's not so much the running of the race that affects your health but the lifestyle changes that often accompany the commitment to run the race. To become a successful runner/marathoner, you need to: (1) follow a proper diet, (2) eliminate extra body fat, (3) refrain from smoking and avoid heavy drinking, (4) get adequate amounts of sleep and (5) exercise regularly. Epidemiologists such as Ralph E. Paffenbarger, M.D., who analyzed the data of Harvard University alumni, have determined that these five lifestyle changes have the potential to add several years to our lives. The marathon lifestyle is definitely a healthy lifestyle.

We have known this at least since the mid-1970s, when the running boom got its start. One of those responsible for projecting marathon running as a healthy activity—or at least not a *dangerous* activity—was T. J. Bassler, M.D., a pathologist at Centinella Valley Community Hospital in California and one of the founders of the American Medical Joggers Association. Dr. Bassler proposed the theory that if you could train for and complete a marathon, you would become immune to death by heart attack for at least six months. He later extended that immunity to a year—then beyond a year.

Dr. Bassler's marathon immunity theory ignited an instant controversy. Many people, including members of the medical establishment, considered his theory not only unfounded but outrageous. A few considered it dangerous because they thought it would lure ill-prepared people to the starting line.

The criticism centered on the fact that Dr. Bassler had no evidence. He had not done a controlled study. All he had done was propose a theory and ask medical experts to prove him wrong— which was not the way serious medical research was conducted.

Over a period of years, eminent cardiologists attempted to dispute Dr. Bassler's theory. They would cite evidence of a runner dead of a heart attack, and Dr. Bassler would point out that the runner didn't run marathons. They would cite a marathoner collapsing in the last mile, and Dr. Bassler would note that the runner didn't finish the race. Dr. Bassler refused to accept anecdotal evidence of coronary deaths, demanding to see x-rays. In several apparent marathon coronary deaths, he identified the culprit as dehydration or a cardiac arrhythmia rather than the standard heart attack caused by blocked arteries. On several occasions, when seemingly pinned into a corner with his theory disproved, Dr. Bassler would modify the theory just enough to maintain the controversy.

On numerous occasions over the years, I had interviewed Dr. Bassler for books and articles and found him almost pixielike. His face was serious, but his eyes twinkled. Although he always professed to be 100 percent committed to his theory of marathon immunity, I was never quite certain whether or not he was serious or merely putting us on.

But he certainly succeeded in convincing the general public that running distances of 26 miles and 385 yards was not fraught with danger, that marathoners were not routinely collapsing, clutching their hearts, that marathon running should not be banned from city streets as a matter of public safety. Each critic of Dr. Bassler, by digging deep to uncover examples of supposed marathon deaths, inadvertently was proving what I consider to be his main message: that marathon running was a relatively safe sport and a benign activity as long as you trained intelligently, behaved rationally and took proper precautions (such as drinking plenty of liquids on hot and humid days).

I'm not sure if cardiologists ever succeeded in disproving the Bassler theory of marathon immunity. More likely, everybody simply lost interest as marathons became a fixture of twentieth-century civilization. By the mid-1980s, a decade after the start of the running boom, enough marathons had been run and enough runners had survived marathons that an occasional cardiac death in a race was considered no more or less alarming than someone dying while attending a football game. Dr. Bassler faded into the backwaters of marathon celebrity, but his immunity theories certainly helped create the marathon mystique.

Bigger and Better

And there definitely is a mystique—no doubt about it. You can run 10-K races until your dresser drawers overflow with T-shirts, but it's not quite the same as going to the starting line of a marathon. "For many runners, it is their personal measuring post and the one distance they want to conquer," says Robert Eslick, a coach from Nashville, Tennessee.

Marathons, on average, seem to be bigger events than races run at shorter distances. Even though more runners turn out for shorter races—such as San Francisco's 12-K Bay-to-Breakers or Spokane, Washington's 12-K Bloomsday Run or Atlanta's 10-K Peachtree Run—marathons *seem* bigger. Witness the excitement attending the big-city marathons: Boston, New York, Chicago, Los Angeles, Twin Cities. Arrive several days in advance of one of those races and you *know* you're at a Big Event, regardless of how many people are entered.

Maybe the excitement is partly anticipation among those entered. Each runner has committed so many miles in training for this one event that the race takes on a level of importance above and beyond the ordinary, regardless of the size of the field. While researching this book, I visited Toledo, Ohio, to lecture the night before the Glass City Marathon, which attracted about 500 runners. Yet despite that relatively small number, the same pre-marathon excitement was present. I could feel it around me as I spoke. People often talk about there being a "glow" around pregnant women. That's certainly true, but there's a similar glow around expectant marathoners. Many of them also have devoted nine months of preparation for their big event. All of those people in my audience at Toledo had worked hard to get ready for the race. Looking at their faces, I envied them.

After my talk, I climbed in my car and drove home to Michigan City, which took me three or four hours and wasn't much fun. But the marathon my audience would run the next morning—also taking three or four hours—*would* be fun. Meanwhile, I had eight more weeks before I would run the marathon I was training for.

What is it about the marathon? Is it the race's history? Its traditions? The many fine runners who have run it? The marathon is all of that, but there's a mystique about the distance itself. Would the race have the same appeal if it were a more logical 25 miles? Or 40 kilometers?

Footsteps of Pheidippides

The establishment of the marathon at the unquestionably odd distance of 26 miles and 385 yards (or 42.2 kilometers) certainly adds to the mystique. The first event to be called a marathon was held in 1896 at the first modern Olympic Games in Athens, Greece. This long-distance footrace was staged at the end of those games to re-create and commemorate the legendary run of Pheidippides in 490 B.C.

In that year, the Persians invaded Greece, landing near the plains of Marathon on Greece's eastern coast. According to the legend, an Athenian general dispatched Pheidippides, a *hemero-dromo,* or runner-messenger, to Sparta (150 miles away) to seek help. Pheidippides reportedly took two days to reach Sparta. The Spartans never did arrive in time to help, but the Athenians eventually overwhelmed their enemy, killing 6,400 Persian troops while losing only 192 of their own men. Or so it was recorded by Greek historians of the time.

Some historians dispute those numbers, suspecting them to be the typically exaggerated claims of the victors. Some historians think Pheidippides may actually have been the messenger dispatched to Athens with news of the victory.

Regardless, Pheidippides supposedly ran a route that took him south along the coast and up and across a series of coastal foothills before descending into Athens, a distance of about 25 miles from the plains of Marathon. According to legend, Pheidippides announced, "Rejoice. We conquer!" as he arrived in Athens—then he fell dead.

Ah, legends. Latter-day historians doubt the total accuracy of the legend, as did the late Jim Fixx, who traced Pheidippides' journey for a *Sports Illustrated* article that became part of *Jim Fixx's Second Book of Running.* If there were a hemerodromo, he may not have been the same one known to have relayed the request for troops to Sparta. There may or may not have been a hemerodromo by that name who died following a postbattle run to Athens. Fixx and others noted that Herodotus, who first described the Battle of Marathon, failed to mention a hemerodromo; the story only appeared four centuries later when retold by Plutarch.

Nevertheless, the legend took on the imprint of historical fact and was certainly no less worthy of respect than legends involving mythical Greek gods such as Hermes or Aphrodite. It seemed perfectly suitable at the 1896 Olympic Games to run a race in Pheidippides' honor from the plains of Marathon to the Olympic stadium in downtown Athens. It was particularly fitting that a Greek shepherd named Spiridon Loues won that event, the only gold medal in track and field won by the Greeks on their home turf.

Among the American clubs represented at those first Games was the Boston Athletic Association, whose team manager was John Graham. So impressed was Graham with this race that he decided to sponsor a similar event in his home town the following year. Races of approximately 25 miles (40 kilometers) had been held before in Europe, including one in France before the Olympics. But nobody had attached the name *marathon* to these races, and there wasn't yet a marathon mystique.

Fifteen runners lined up at the start of the first Boston Marathon in 1897 to race from suburban Hopkinton into downtown Boston, and a new legend was born. Since the Olympic marathon is run only every fourth year, Boston remains the oldest continuously held marathon. It continues to retain its status and prestige despite bigger and richer events held around the world each year. (A previous American marathon was run in the fall of 1896 from Stamford, Connecticut, to Columbus Circle, near the finish line of the current New York City Marathon, but it failed to survive.)

Determining the Distance

For a dozen years, the official marathon distance remained approximately 25 miles. That was the distance run in the 1900 Paris Olympic Games and the 1904 St. Louis games. Then in 1908, in London, the British designed a marathon course that started at Windsor Castle and finished at the Olympic stadium. This was in an era long before course certification experts measured race distances to an accuracy of plus or minus a few feet. Nobody challenged the British course design, which reportedly was laid out to let the royal family see the start of the race.

The distance from start to finish in that 1908 Olympic marathon was precisely 26 miles and 385 yards. For whatever reason, that distance became the standard for future marathons. Frank Shorter tells the story of running the marathon trials for the 1971 Pan American Games. At 21 miles, he was lockstep with Kenny Moore, a 1968 Olympian. "Why couldn't Pheidippides have died here," Shorter groaned to Moore. In this case, it was Shorter who "died" and Moore who went on to win the race.

The event that is so popular today might not be the same if the plains of Marathon had been closer to Athens. Exercise physiologists tell us that it is only after about two hours of running— or about 20 miles for an accomplished runner—that the body begins to fully deplete its stores of glycogen, the energy source that fuels the muscles. Once glycogen is depleted, the body must rely more on fat, a less efficient fuel source. This is one of the reasons runners hit the "Wall" at 20 miles, and successfully getting past that obstacle is what makes the marathon such a special event.

Many of us who consider ourselves accomplished runners— and who are well trained—run 20-milers as part of our weekly training regimen without excessive pain and with little fanfare. It is only when we stretch beyond that point that people sit up and take notice. Would a million people line the roads at the Boston and New York City marathons if the distance were only 20 miles and if there were no Wall to conquer? No, they want to see us tempt the fate of Pheidippides. They come to see us suffer, although inevitably both spectator and runner leave fulfilled only if we demonstrate through our successful crashing through the Wall and crossing of the finish line (regardless of our time) that we are victorious.

Changing Your Life

For many, completing one marathon is enough. It changes their lives forever. Professional photographers who take pictures of runners crossing the finish line find that two or three times as many people order prints of their marathon finishes, compared to runners who finish shorter races. It's the same reason that people order more pictures at weddings. It's an extra special event. It's like tacking a Ph.D. at the end of your name, getting married, having a baby. You're special, whether anyone else knows it or not. You certainly do. Your life will never again be quite the same, and regardless of what the future brings, you can look back and say, "I finished a marathon." Others consider it a continuing challenge of numbers: personal records (or PRs), which exist to be bettered at each race. Even when inevitable declines in performance accompany aging, new challenges arise as the lifetime marathoner moves from one five-year bracket to another.

It is also possible to run marathons recreationally, not caring about time or finishing position but participating merely for the joy of attending a great event with all its accompanying pleasures. I have run many marathons in this manner, running within myself and finishing far back from where I might have, had I pushed the pace harder.

One year at the Honolulu Marathon, I started in the back row and made a game out of passing as many people as possible—but doing it at a pace barely faster than theirs so as not to call attention to my speed, so it didn't seem that I was trying to show them up. I've also run marathons with planned dropout points, using the race as a workout to prepare for later marathons. At the World Veterans Championships in Rome in 1985, I ran the marathon at the end of a week's track competition mainly so I could enjoy the sights and sounds of the Eternal City. Entering a piazza in the last miles of the race with a panoramic view across the Tiber River of St. Peter's Cathedral, I paused for several minutes to absorb that view, then continued toward the stadium used for the 1960 Olympic Games. How fast I ran, or how well I placed, were the last things on my mind.

Crossing the finish line, more refreshed than fatigued, I was approached by an Australian runner, who announced, "This is the first time I ever beat you."

I felt obliged to correct him: "You didn't beat me. You merely finished in front of me."

The Australian stammered an apology, but he had missed the point of the marathon. Or at least the marathon the way I had chosen to run it that particular day. In the marathon, you don't beat others, as you might in a mile or a 100-meter dash. Instead, you achieve a personal victory. If others finish in front of or behind you, it is only that their personal victories are more or less. A person finishing behind you with lesser talent, or a different age, or sex, or various other limiting factors, may have achieved a far greater victory than yours. At the 1992 Boston Marathon, John A. Kelley, age 84, finished in a time of 5:58:32. The officials stopped timing at five hours, at which point 8,120 runners had crossed the line (not counting those running unofficially without numbers). It was the 61st and final time "Old John," a two-time winner of the race, would run Boston. None of the thousands finishing in front of Kelley could be said to have beaten him. He is a legend—like Pheidippides.

One beauty of the marathon is that there are many more winners than those who finish first overall or in their age groups. "Everyone's a winner" is a dreadful cliché, but it happens to be true when the race involved is 26 miles and 385 yards long.

A Lifetime of Marathons

Reporters sometimes ask how many marathons I have run. My pat answer is, "About a hundred."

This amazes them: "You've run 100 marathons?"

I have to correct them, because I don't want to see in the newspaper the next morning that I have finished marathon number 101. "No," I say. "I don't know how many marathons I've run. But it must be about a hundred."

That doesn't satisfy reporters with statistical fixations, but I've been telling reporters "about a hundred" for the last ten years. The true number could be less, but most likely it is more.

Sy Mah, the Toledo, Ohio, runner who often ran two and sometimes three marathons on a weekend, finished 524 races longer than 26 miles before his death from cancer at age 62 in 1988. That was the focal point of Mah's running, so it was important that he keep precise records for each of his races. He was another legend.

Mah usually finished in the high three-hour range. I once told him that if he focused his attention for six months on a single race—training specifically for it, resisting the temptation to run other marathons and tapering and peaking—he could probably improve his time by a half hour, and maybe even break three hours, putting him near the top of his age group. Smiling, he conceded my point, but we both knew that was not what he was about. His joy was running as many marathons as possible and adding to his impressive string of numbers, which had earned him an enviable spot in *The Guinness Book of World Records.*

In comparison, my own stunt during the fall of 1991 in running six marathons in six weekends at the age of 60 was trivial, almost inconsequential. My six, even my lifetime number of "about a hundred," was merely a blip on the chart compared to the 524 marathons finished by Sy Mah.

Despite sore and aching muscles, despite dehydration and fatigue, despite the apparent disgrace of having been beaten soundly by runners who normally would finish far behind me, there were moments of joy in each of those half dozen marathons. As there were moments of joy in each of the "about a hundred" other marathons I had run in a career spanning nearly a half century.

It is only because the marathon never ceases to be a race of joy, a race of wonder. Even when disaster strikes, when bad weather overwhelms you, when an intemperate pace results in a staggering finish, when nerves and anxiety impede a maximum effort, when your number one rival soundly thrashes you, when nine months of training appears to have gone down the drain with little more than an ugly slurping sound, there remains something memorable about each marathon run.

I would have a hard time explaining that to the woman beside the course at the Twin Cities Marathon, who considered it odd that we actually had paid to "abuse" our bodies. But anyone who has crossed the finish line of a 26-mile, 385-yard race would understand. Sy Mah knew. It's all part of the magic of the marathon.

CHAPTER 2

A Word to the
BEGINNING
RUNNER

People need not be taught how to run. Children learn to run almost as soon as they learn to walk. Visit any elementary school playground, and you'll see kids sprinting all over the place. All children are born sprinters.

Children modify their behavior as they get older. Running starts to become a discipline rather than a natural form of exercise. An athlete who goes out for any sport in high school—football, basketball, tennis or whatever—runs as part of the conditioning for that sport. High schoolers run either because their coach told them to or because they know getting in shape will help them make the team. Usually, young athletes run middle distance: a few laps on a track, then off to the main activity. It is only as adults that people forget to run and sometimes have to be retaught.

Let's talk about being a beginning runner. If you're an experienced runner who trains regularly and competes in 10-K races, you probably could skip this chapter. With one or two exceptions, it probably won't teach you anything you don't already know. But maybe you'd like to look over my shoulder as I talk to beginning runners and get them started on their first journeys.

Before you can hope to run long distances, you must start by

running short—and running slowly. Some beginners (particularly if they're overweight) need to walk first, beginning with a half
hour, three or four days a week. Then they jog a short distance
until they get slightly out of breath, walk to recover, jog some
more. Jog, walk. Jog, walk. Jog, walk. After a while, they can run
a mile without stopping.

Before we move forward, there are some important kernels of
information hidden in the paragraph above. Even experienced
runners can learn from it.

The pattern is: Jog, *walk.* Jog, *walk.* Jog, *walk.* Expressed
another way: Hard, *easy.* Hard, *easy.* Hard, *easy.* The most effective training programs—even at the basic level—mix bursts of
difficult training with rest. Train, *rest.* Train, *rest.* Train, *rest.*

Rest. That may be the single most important word you will
read in this book. (You'll encounter it again and again.) In the
questionnaire I sent to coaches, one of the questions was: "How
important is rest in the training equation?"

The very first coach to return a completed questionnaire was
Paul Goss of Foster City, California. His response was simple
and direct: "More important than most runners know."

None of the more than 50 other coaches who eventually
responded improved on what Goss had to say.

Learning to Run

With beginners the problem is not to get them to rest but to
get them to *stop* resting. They have to get off the couch and away
from the TV. They must learn to become participants in sport,
rather than spectators of sport. To those of us who accept running as a natural activity, that's not as easy as it might seem.

Beginners need motivation to begin—and to keep at it once
they have begun. "The key factor in any beginner's training program is motivation," suggests Jack Daniels, Ph.D., exercise physiologist and coach at the State University of New York in
Cortland. "If you're genetically gifted but not interested in training, you'll never develop."

Barring some medical problem, most people can run, but they
aren't motivated to do so. Even if they want to start running, it
takes courage to put on running shoes and step out on a side-

walk for the first time in view of friends and neighbors. A lot of potential runners never get moving out of fear of looking foolish. They lack self-confidence. They fear failure.

It sometimes helps to join a class. One advantage of a class situation is the group support you get from others of equal ability or lack of ability. The most important information any coach can offer beginners is not how to hold their arms, or how far to jog without stopping, but simply, "You're looking good. You're doing great. Keep it up." Basic motivation. Natural running instincts, overlooked but not forgotten from childhood, will take over.

Joining a class can provide you with support, information and good training routes, but particularly with motivation as you train with friends. If you are looking for a running class in your area, check with local health clubs, running clubs, sporting goods stores or the organizers of major races. One good source of information is the Road Runners Club of America (RRCA, 629 South Washington Street, Alexandria, VA 22314; 703-836-0558), which has 490 member clubs with 150,000 members. The RRCA can point you in the right direction if you're looking to connect with other runners and runner support groups.

Many books also have been written on beginning running. Jim Fixx's *The Complete Book of Running,* which sold nearly a million copies in the United States alone, got many people started running. Most books and classes for beginners provide similar advice: Begin at an easy level; don't try to do too much too soon; don't get discouraged when your muscles ache.

And don't focus immediately upon the marathon. "Too many runners attempt the marathon far too early in their careers and then become ex-runners," notes Robert Eslick, a coach from Nashville, Tennessee. When asked how long it should take a beginning runner to train for and complete a marathon, our panel of coaches concurred that most people could do so in just over a year. Some might take more time, some less. Asked how long experienced runners should train for a marathon, most coaches suggested a training period about half as long. (The actual figures, when averaged, were 13.38 months for novices and 7.26 months for experienced runners.)

But before beginning to think about running a marathon, you first need to think about beginning running.

Checking Out the System

People older than 35 who want to start exercising should consider having a medical examination, including an exercise stress test. The American College of Sports Medicine recommends testing at age 40 for men and age 50 for women—if you're apparently healthy. But if you have any risk factor for coronary artery disease (high blood pressure, high cholesterol, smoking, diabetes or family history of heart problems), testing should be done prior to vigorous exercise, for *any* age.

"This is particularly important if your family has a history of heart disease," states Jack Scaff, Jr., M.D., one of the founders of the Honolulu Marathon. "If you have been overweight or recently were a smoker, your risks also are high." Running is a relatively safe activity, but why take a chance?

The cardiology departments of many major medical centers provide exercise stress tests for around $250, often covered by health insurance. The best type of test is "symptom-limited," in which you exercise until you attain your maximum heart rate, unless symptoms develop. A cardiologist uses an electrocardiograph (EKG) to monitor heartbeat while you walk or jog on a treadmill. Or they may test you pedaling an ergometer (exercise bicycle). The cardiologist will also record blood pressure. If your coronary arteries are even partially blocked, it should become apparent during stress. Changes in your heartbeat will appear on the EKG screen and you will be asked to stop.

This does not mean you cannot run, but you will need to begin under careful medical supervision. Doctors regularly prescribe exercise, including running, for patients who have suffered heart attacks. It is not uncommon for heart attack victims to eventually finish marathons.

If no symptoms develop during your exam—and assuming there are no other medical problems—you will be cleared to start running.

Just because you pass an exercise stress test once, however, that's no guarantee you will never suffer a heart attack, either while running or while engaged in other activities. Physicians now recommend you have a physical every two or three years, more often as you get older or if your cardiologist determines you're in a high-risk category. Also, learn the heart attack symptoms. The classic symptoms include chest pain, but symptoms can include *any* generalized pain between the eyeballs and the belly button, even a toothache. "It's a myth that tingling occurs only in the left arm," says Dr. Scaff. "It can appear in the right arm, too." If such symptoms develop during a run, stop running immediately and seek medical advice. Even if the symptoms seem to diminish as you continue to run, that doesn't mean you're safe.

How to Begin

If you've never run before, focus your attention on time rather than distance or pace. Put on a pair of comfortable shoes. While you will eventually need running shoes, for your first couple of short outings you can start with whatever you have.

Start to jog gently, on a grassy or dirt surface if possible. Jog until you're somewhat out of breath, then begin to walk. Resume jogging when you feel comfortable, walking again if necessary. "Most people overestimate what they can do," says Stan James, M.D., an orthopedist from Eugene, Oregon. When your tired muscles won't let you jog any more, finish by walking. Set as your goal 15 minutes of combined jogging and walking.

Record your time in a diary or simply on your calendar. Don't worry about distance and pace this early in your training.

Take the next day off. On the third day, repeat the first day's workout, but again don't worry about distance. If you go much farther or faster than the first day, you may be progressing too rapidly. Take the fourth day off.

On the fifth day, again repeat the basic workout, then rest the sixth and seventh days. Your training has followed the classic hard/easy pattern used by former University of Oregon track coach Bill Bowerman and countless other top coaches in training world-class runners. The pattern is the same; only the degree of difficulty is different.

The second week, simply repeat the workouts you did during the first week. You may feel that you can run farther or go faster, but hold back. When Bowerman developed his championship athletes at the University of Oregon, he always felt it was better

that they be somewhat *undertrained* rather than *overtrained.*
Even though there was a chance the Oregon athletes might perform slightly below their potential while undertrained, their
chances for injury were greatly reduced. If that conservative
approach made sense for his highly talented athletes, why
shouldn't it also work for you?

The second week is critical in any beginning running program.
You may have been able to run through week one just from sheer
beginner's enthusiasm. Even if your muscles were sore, running
seemed harder than you expected, and you failed to see any
improvement, you probably were able to keep going from the
momentum generated by your decision to begin.

But now you're into your second week. Maybe your muscles
are still sore, you're getting bored with the same every-other-day
routine, and it's dawned on you that you probably will never win
an Olympic gold medal. You haven't yet experienced that "runner's high" one of your friends promised you. And it may feel as if
running will never get any better.

Hang in there; it will.

Continuing to Run

Beginning with week three, and continuing through weeks
four, five and six, add three minutes to your workout each seven
days. During a six-week beginner's training period, your daily
and weekly (based on three workout days) training mileage
should be as follows:

Week	Time per Day (minutes)	Time per Week (minutes)
1	15	45
2	15	45
3	18	54
4	21	63
5	24	72
6	27	81

How fast should you be running? It doesn't matter. You should only be worrying about time, not distance or pace. You can record those variables, but if you try to increase your mileage and your pace, you're more likely to get injured. Better to go too slow in the beginning than too fast.

At the end of this initial six-week training period, treat yourself to a half-hour run. When finished, consider what you have accomplished. In a period of six weeks, you have *doubled* your initial workout load. As you continue to run, there will be few times when you will be able to improve at this rate: 100 percent improvement in only six weeks! Improvement comes easily and suddenly when you're a beginner. It's more difficult for more experienced runners and *incredibly* difficult for those at the top of the performance charts. But you should continue to improve as a runner for many months, and perhaps years to come, as long as you follow a sensible training program.

Moving Up the Training Ladder

Almost all training designed to improve runners is based on moving from level to level. You work harder and improve, moving from a low level to a higher level. This is your body's progressive adaptation to increasing stress.

Different coaches have different approaches when it comes to teaching runners how to improve, how to move from one level to the next and how to turn a beginner into an experienced runner. One of the challenges given to the coaches who received my questionnaire was to devise marathon training programs for first-time runners, experienced runners and elite runners. The question was: "What should this runner do on a day-by-day basis, midseason?"

Seven of the coaches who responded to my questionnaire also supplied training programs designed for first-time, experienced, and elite marathoners, which are presented in chapter 17. Naturally there are limits to how hard you can train and how much you can improve. Not everybody can move from the first level in these training programs through the second and then to the third—and just moving to the second level may provide all the challenge you need. But even genetically gifted athletes need time to move from level to level to level. If you overtrain, you're likely to crash. Even if you don't injure yourself, you may discover that your competitive efforts deteriorate. You begin to run slower instead of faster.

Sooner or later, this happens to almost all top athletes. According to Dick Brown, the former Athletics West coach from Eugene, Oregon, "Most of the time, athletes need to be held back rather than pushed."

Top athletes are constantly pressing against the "edge of the envelope," trying to measure the limits of human performance. "There are two ways to learn about training," states Dr. James, the orthopedist from Oregon. "One is by having access to a very knowledgeable coach. The other is by trial and error." With a knowledgeable coach, errors result less frequently.

But if you are an athlete working without a coach, you may have difficulty recognizing how much and how fast to run. "Most people mis-estimate what they do," says Dr. James. "There is a difference between what the body perceives and what the mind perceives."

The 5 Percent Solution

How can you maximize your performance? How much can you improve?

When asked how much improvement runners might expect following a year's hard training, Dr. Jack Daniels suggests 5 percent as an upper limit. But it's a tough question. "There is no physiological basis for saying how much you can increase your workload," Dr. Daniels finally admits. Runners differ enormously in both their capability and capacity, says Dr. Daniels: "Some people with little training background have tremendous potential for improvement. Others who have been running for many years may have improved as much as they can."

A new runner capable of running a 10-K in 50:00 may find it relatively easy to improve by 5 percent, which would mean cutting 2½ minutes to improve to 47:30. A similar 5 percent improvement for a runner capable of running a 10-K in 30:00 would be somewhat less: 1½ minutes, or 28:30. However, few athletes improve that much at that performance level without many years of increased training—and maybe not even then.

So if you can improve by 5 percent, you can be said to have outperformed the world's elite. That should be sufficient motivation to get you moving. Most average runners, however, would settle for a 1 percent improvement, which would allow someone who runs a 10-K in 40:00 to get down to 39:36.

Four Key Performance Factors

Anyone can improve with practice, says Dr. Daniels. "Where you start, and whether or not you are genetically gifted, dictates where you finish—provided you optimize what you have," he says. "Optimizing what you have is the tricky part."

Dr. Daniels suggests four areas in which runners improve in ability.

1. **Oxygen delivery.** When the heart muscle becomes stronger, your oxygen delivery system becomes more efficient.

2. **Oxygen absorption.** Training also results in increased blood flow through the muscle fibers and improvement of the fibers themselves—all of which improves your ability to use oxygen.

3. **Economy.** You can learn to run faster while expending the same amount of energy by improving technique and form.

4. **Endurance.** This means increasing how fast you can run before you hit your pain threshold. Basically, stronger muscles contract more effectively.

To improve to the highest level requires talent. But even those of average talent can rise above their abilities and achieve extremely high levels of success as runners. In perhaps no event is this more true than the marathon.

CHAPTER 3

Your First
MARATHON

S now fluttering in the air. Temperature 20°. Cold wind from the north.
Ron Gunn, who coaches runners at Southwestern Michigan
College, said his team had almost frozen during their afternoon
workout.

Still, it wasn't a bad night for a run. It was a Thursday in mid-
March, the first night of a class to prepare for the Sunburst
Marathon in South Bend, Indiana, in June. Gunn regularly
teaches running classes in the area around South Bend, and his
graduates have run marathons around the world.

Because of the weather, only 15 showed for our first session. It
seemed ironic that we would begin in such cold to prepare for a
June race that, despite a 6:00 A.M. start, historically has suffered
from heat and humidity, conditions not always conducive to fast
times. But as a marathoner, I accept conditions as they come—
either in training or in races.

Thus, I didn't consider it a bad night for a run.

Running with Friends

After a brief classroom session, we climbed in the "Green
Gorilla," the affectionate name bestowed on the green-painted
school bus Gunn uses to transport his team and classes. We
drove to near the bridge over the St. Joseph's River in Niles,
Michigan, just across the Indiana-Michigan state line. We
planned to run south along the river, with the wind at our backs.

When we arrived at the bridge, a pair of cyclists were readying their trail bikes for a ride along the same route. The weather didn't discourage them, either.

The cyclists pedaled away and we started after them downriver. I began at the back and worked up through the pack, asking people their names. There was Bill and Harry and Geoff and Tim. A woman said her name was "Alloyed—like in steel." She was moving fast, so I ran with her. Another runner had darted ahead. We caught him when he stopped at a corner, unsure which way to turn, then he darted off again.

The river road was dirt, then pavement pitted with potholes, then dirt again. Gunn greeted us with a jug of water balanced on the fender of the bus. I knew we'd be particularly happy for his support as Sunburst got nearer and the weather warmed.

It was soon dark. Traffic along the road was sporadic. Most drivers moved over when their headlights flashed on our reflective clothing. But one switched his lights on bright and almost forced us off the road. I heard him honking at the others behind to get out of his way. Some people are jerks, and some people run marathons.

One reason I decided to teach a class with Ron that spring was to bring me in touch with real runners. I talk to world-class athletes all the time, but that's not the real runner's world. I figured I'd learn as much from the class as they would from me. But a greater goal was to use class support to train harder. I had set my goal that spring as breaking three hours at Sunburst, a time I had not achieved for some years. One of the ways to achieve enjoyment as a runner is to set goals, and one of the ways to succeed in your goals is to join a class, either as student or teacher. Or as Tim told me while we ran shoulder-to-shoulder that evening, "I run harder when I run with friends."

Differing Goals

There are three goals in marathon running: to finish, to improve and to win. Which goal you strive for depends on what level of running you're at.

To finish is important to the beginning runner. To cover 26 miles and 385 yards equals victory. Regardless of time, regardless of place, the prime goal is to get to the finish line standing up and in reasonably good shape. And to enjoy the experience! Regardless of how fast or slow you finish—unless you set your goals too high—you will look on that first completed marathon as a significant experience, a portentous point in your life.

Whether or not you, as a first-time marathoner, *enjoy* the experience enough to become a next-time marathoner may be irrelevant. For most beginners, to finish is to win. And for many, once is enough.

To improve is the goal of the seasoned runner. "Seasoned" could describe anybody who has been running several years, has finished his or her first marathon—or two or three—and now wants to run faster. Improving from six hours to five, from five hours to four, from four hours to three, or various gradients within those hour blocks is akin to victory. Setting personal records is the name of the game for many of us. It doesn't matter if the PR is for your career, your current age group, the year or the month of June. Take your victories where you can find them.

Improvement doesn't come easily. You have to work at it. If you finished your first marathon by training 35 miles a week, you may need to increase your mileage to 45 or 55, or more, to improve in future marathons. You may need to add speedwork and other means of fine-tuning your skills (or compensating for lack of skills). You may need to add supplemental exercises, lift weights and learn to stretch properly to get better. You also may need to pay attention to diet. Prerace diet is particularly important in endurance events lasting over two hours, as is fluid intake.

At some point in each marathoner's life, it becomes increasingly difficult to snip seconds off your PR. And inevitably, if you stay in marathoning long enough, improvement may become impossible—at least as measured on the clock.

Nevertheless, each move to a new (five-year) age group permits improvement within that age group. And as an aging runner's career passes peaks and valleys, it is possible to allow yourself to sink to new lows (by backing off training) so that you can establish new highs (by increasing that training). For some runners, every marathon is like their first one, each one a new adventure. I certainly feel that way, and I don't consider myself unique. Depending upon how you view the sport, you can continue to improve as a marathoner forever.

To win is the goal of the elite runner, but winning is something only a small percentage of runners will ever achieve. In my long career encompassing more than 100 marathon races, I've won at least three overall: Windy City in Chicago in 1964; Heart of America in Columbus, Missouri, in 1968; and Longest Day in Brookings, South Dakota, in 1972. I may have won one or two more that I've forgotten about, and I've won my age group on numerous occasions, including a TAC (The Athletics Congress) national age-group championship and a $250 cash prize at the 1991 Twin Cities Marathon.

My early wins came relatively easily. Decades ago in the United States, the typical road race attracted at best a few dozen runners. If you were a reasonably competent runner, the odds were decent that you might cross the finish line in first place. My three victories above were with times slower than 2:30, pedestrian by today's standards.

In today's marathon scene, with race fields as large as 25,000 and first place cash prizes of $50,000 or more, the odds of crossing the line first have diminished considerably. Fewer than 1 percent of those running—much fewer—have a chance of crossing a finish line first. A slightly larger percentage might earn an award for finishing high in their age group. Most people return from a completed marathon with no more than a race T-shirt and a medal or certificate given to all finishers.

Nevertheless, the training secrets that work for the running elite—the ones whose pictures appear on the cover of *Runner's World,* if not *Rolling Stone*—can be applied to allow the less gifted to improve and maximize their potential. And this itself may be a more significant victory than merely crossing the finish line first.

Boston: A Favorite Goal

One standard of achievement is running fast enough to qualify for the Boston Marathon, the granddaddy of American marathons. When I first ran Boston in 1959, anyone could enter—and there wasn't even an entry fee! Fewer than 200 of us appeared that Patriot's Day. Within the decade, however, the

Boston race had become so popular that organizers imposed a qualifying time of four hours to limit the field.

That merely spurred runners to train harder. Boston became *the* standard for marathon excellence. By qualifying for the Boston Marathon, runners achieved status among their peers. It earned you bragging rights to be able to say nonchalantly that you had "qualified for Boston." Boston's numbers continued to increase, because once a runner qualified, it seemed almost obligatory to go to Boston to run. So organizers of the marathon kept lowering the standard until by the mid-1980s, if you were a man under 40 you had to break 2:50 to qualify.

That made the standard almost too tough. Three hours was a reasonable time for a runner of average ability who was willing to train hard over a period of years, but to go ten minutes under that time requires a certain natural ability. To get into Boston, you needed to combine talent and training.

Eventually, Boston relaxed its standards to 3:00 for the fastest age group with a sliding scale of slower times in other categories depending upon age and sex. To qualify in 1993, you had to run faster than 3:10 on a certified course if you were a man younger than 35. Beyond that age, the standard relaxed five minutes every five years: 3:15 for age 35, 3:20 for age 40, etc. The base standard for women is 3:40 with a similar sliding upward scale.

Actually, most studies on aging suggest that sedentary people lose fitness at the rate of about 1 percent a year, which is 10 percent a decade. Most runners who maintain their training probably decline at a lesser rate, perhaps 0.5 percent a year, 5 percent a decade. So as runners continue in the sport, it becomes easier and easier to qualify for the Boston Marathon. A time of 3:30 for a man aged 50 or a time of 4:00 for a woman age 50 is within reach of most readers of this book—if they're willing to devote a decade of their lives to attaining it. For that reason, a majority of the field at Boston is masters runners, over age 40.

What to Aim For

The first rule for anyone starting his or her first marathon, unless you are among the running elite mentioned above, is to make your goal merely finishing the race. Select a pace and shoot for a time much slower than you think possible just to get a finish under your belt. After achieving the "victory" of a finish, then—and only then—should you contemplate training harder to finish with faster times.

Almost anyone can finish a marathon. The distance is 26 miles and 385 yards, not that far when you think about it. Merely by walking at a comfortable pace of three miles an hour, you could cover it in about nine hours. Not many people would be waiting around to greet you, but you could finish.

By jogging a bit, or even walking somewhat faster, you can finish in a slightly better time. The last-place finisher in the Honolulu Marathon, one of the few races where the officials wait for everybody, usually comes in at around eight or nine hours. By jogging and walking, you should be able to move at a speed of four miles an hour. That will get you to the finish line in under seven hours.

In 1983, my wife, Rose, took a year's sabbatical from her work as a teacher to research her family history. I was leading a tour of runners to the Honolulu Marathon and said (somewhat maliciously) that I'd take her, but only if she ran the race. She said okay, trained a bit in addition to her tennis, biking and other activities, and finished the marathon in 6½ hours, walking a good portion of the second half. I bought her a special plaque commemorating what she still considers a special achievement— although she has no plans to run another marathon.

Several years later, our daughter Laura trained hard enough to knock an hour off the family female time at the Chicago Marathon. I ran with Laura, who walked a lot in the closing stages and finished in better shape than I did. Slow running is not necessarily easier than fast running. Four-time Boston and New York City marathon champion Bill Rodgers once said respectfully about those in the back of the pack, "I can't even imagine what it's like to run for five or six hours."

With a little more conditioning and determination, however, you can run at a 12-minute-per-mile pace, or 5 miles per hour. This allows you to complete the marathon distance in close to five hours, which is a reasonable goal for a "fitness jogger" who wants only to finish. In most of the big marathons today, many people cross the line at around five hours, smiling proudly, looking and feeling better than many of those who preceded them in half that time.

Moving into the four-hour or three-hour bracket requires more training, however, and getting into the two-hour bracket requires both training and talent. The world record for men is currently 2:06:50 by Belayne Densimo of Ethiopia, and we may be years away from seeing a runner break two hours and move into the one-hour bracket. Some pundits believe we will *never* see that day—although I can remember when the world record was in the mid 2:20s. Great Britain's Jim Peters, who has been described as the greatest marathoner ever, improved the world record from 2:26:07 to 2:17:39 between 1952 and 1954.

In that era, less than a half century ago, many considered a sub-2:20 marathon nearly impossible, but we have been required to revise our thinking about the limits of human achievement. The women's marathon record is 2:21:06, held by Norway's Ingrid Kristiansen. At one point, female runners were restricted to races of a few miles, because male officials believed them incapable of going much farther. Try telling that to Ingrid!

Impossible goals sometimes prove possible. Most people, of course, never come close to achieving the times of the running elite. At the 1991 Boston Marathon, the median time was 3:18:24 for men, 3:41:28 for women, which means that half the field finished faster and half finished slower. Boston, however, attracts a semi-elite field, because of its time standards. The New York City Marathon, however, accepts entrants regardless of past marathon performances, and at the 1991 race the median times were 3:58:27 for men and 4:29:14 for women. The New York data is probably typical for most marathons, says Basil Honikman of TACSTATS. This means that if you want to rise above average, the goal for a man should be 4:00 and for a woman, 4:30.

At the bottom of the scale, some finishers at the New York City, Los Angeles and Honolulu marathons that same year finished slower than ten hours. The slowest was at Honolulu, where one man took longer than 29 hours! (He fell, was injured, went to the hospital and returned the following day to finish.)

Although statisticians find it convenient to talk about median or average times, I like to believe that there are no average runners. I consider us all *above* average—at least as individuals. When you even begin to consider the possibility of finishing your first marathon, you move well beyond anything that might be described as "average."

Time as a goal becomes irrelevant for someone attempting a marathon. The only goal worth considering for first-time marathoners is the finish line.

Choosing Your First Marathon

Selecting your first marathon may be a critical decision. Unless you decide to run a small, local marathon because it is near home (a logical reason), you probably are best served by entering one of the big-city marathons. With more people in the field, you will feel less lonely running back in the pack, and there usually is more crowd support. If you never have felt loved before, you should try running one of the big-city marathons with spectators lining the course from start to finish, cheering everyone, slow or fast.

In fact, the back-of-the-packers get most of the cheers. Because they're moving slower, they take a longer time to pass those applauding. Often, the leaders dart by so quickly, spectators just stare in awe. It is a sad commentary on the popularity of running that most spectators know little about who is leading the race.

Don Kardong, a senior writer for *Runner's World,* once covered the Boston Marathon from his hotel room. The day before the race, he had scouted the course and written down the telephone numbers of pay phone booths at various intervals. At the proper moment, he would call each booth and ask whoever answered for a report on what he saw. "Who's leading?" he asked one person who answered.

"Just a minute," said the respondent, noting that the lead pack had not yet passed the booth. When he returned to the booth, he announced, "Some cop on a motorcycle."

So no one should feel embarrassed at running far in the rear. Another advantage of a big field is that if you stand in the back row, it may take you several minutes to even cross the starting line, thus removing any latent desire for a fast time. With any luck, the field will be so big that the beginner also will be forced to cover the first several miles at a walk or a very slow jog, thus storing energy for the last few miles.

At the Motor City Marathon in Detroit in 1991, I decided to do just that. With a field of about 2,000 and a wide starting area, it took me about a minute to reach and cross the starting line. I was last of the starting group across the line, although several runners who must have arrived late soon passed me. I walked most of the first mile before eventually breaking into a gentle jog, but I ran the second half of the race faster than the first and finished comfortably—or at least as comfortable as finishing 26 miles can be.

It's an intelligent approach to running the marathon—one, I admit, that I don't always take.

Another reason to run big marathons, at least that first time, is that they often are better financed, with better support systems and more volunteers, resulting in more aid stations and everything else you need to make your race more enjoyable. Not to be overlooked is the glitz and glamour that surrounds many big-city events. Bands playing and balloons in the air may not make you run faster, but it makes you feel better.

A Lesson about Speed

Many marathoners probably could learn a lesson from beginners. Having completed one or two marathons comfortably, though relatively untrained, they often get caught in the trap of thinking that faster is better, that they have to run each race progressively speedier to justify time spent in training. They forget the first marathoner's joy. But sometimes you have to return to your roots by running *slower* than your potential. Realistically speaking, few will know or care whether you fail to run a PR.

One important word of advice: Run your first marathon very slowly. Don't just start slowly, but continue to run slowly. By running your first marathon very slowly, you leave enough room for improvement so that you can take hours, not merely minutes, off your time as you progress from beginning runner to seasoned runner.

As with other endeavors, it is a basic tenet of marathon running that rewards come to those who persevere. We all begin with various levels of talent, but we improve in relation to the amount of effort we expend and how we maximize that talent.

The minimal amount of training for those wishing merely to finish a marathon seems to be around 35 miles a week. The coaches surveyed for this book suggested an average of 35½ miles weekly as the appropriate training mileage for first-time marathoners. That permits a long run of 10 to 15 miles on the weekend and 4- to 5-mile runs the rest of the week, with occasional days off. This works out to maybe a six-hour weekly commitment. For beginners, no speedwork or exotic training regimen featuring various combinations of fartlek, intervals and repeats is necessary—just ordinary slogging down the street. On such slender commitments marathons are finished these days, but not without a certain amount of discomfort, however.

To improve, the beginning runner need only gradually increase the length of the daily runs, which he or she can do without strain as long as the increase is gradual. Over a period of months, the 10- to 15-mile run on the weekend becomes a 15- to 20-mile run. One or two workouts a week may go from 4 to 5, to 6 to 7, then 8 to 10. Almost before realizing it, the beginning runner is covering 50 to 60 miles a week. (Our coach's survey came up with an average of 56½ miles as the mileage necessary for those hoping to improve their times to "finish well.")

Improvement in your marathon times will come relative to increase in mileage—at least to a point.

But the essential goal is to *finish* your first marathon. The expert in that area is a former semipro ice hockey player from Minneapolis, Minnesota, named Bill Wenmark. In the next chapter, I'll tell you about him, beginning with Grandma's Marathon.

CHAPTER 4

The Man Who Coached
1,000
MARATHONERS

One of the questions asked of the coaches consulted for this book was to list, in order, their ten favorite marathons. The response was somewhat predictable, with Boston and New York topping the list, but I was surprised to see one marathon from what was apparently a small town in New England rank in the top ten.

At least it must have been a small town, because I had never heard of it, nor of the race. Jonathan Tiedeman, the member of my cross-country team who had collated results of the questionnaires, had the town listed as *Grand, Mass.*

After puzzling over the list for a minute, I suddenly recognized Jonathan's mistake. It wasn't a small town in New England but rather a small town in Minnesota: Duluth. The race was *Grandma's* Marathon!

I suppose that Jonathan, a high school freshman in his first year of competition, can be excused for looking at "Grandma's" on a bunch of returned questionnaires and mistaking it for a town in Massachusetts. If you are new to running, have not yet completed your first marathon and have purchased this book for some tips to help get you to the finish line, you might make a similar mistake of misidentification.

But Grandma's Marathon has particular significance for many

More about Grandma's

For the record, Grandma's Marathon is usually held the second or third weekend of June in Duluth, Minnesota. The race is point-to-point; it begins near the town of Two Harbors on the northern shore of Lake Superior and follows that shore southwest into Duluth, finishing near the restaurant that served as the main sponsor for the race's first decade: Grandma's Saloon & Deli. And, of course, that's where the race gets its unusual name.

Grandma's Marathon began in 1977 and achieved almost instant celebrity because of fast times by several top Minnesota runners. Garry Bjorklund ran 2:10:20 in 1980, and Dick Beardsley bettered that the next year with a 2:09:37. Lorraine Moeller, a New Zealand runner who trained in Minnesota, set a women's best of 2:29:36 in 1981.

Those fast times attracted more fast runners—and slow runners hoping to become fast runners. During the peak of the running boom, race director Scott Keenan had to limit entrants to 4,500, a number usually achieved within weeks after entry blanks were mailed in January, five months before the race date.

Grandma's numbers lately have plateaued around 5,500, but the race remains popular, partly because its late-spring date permits more preparation time for runners in the upper Midwest. Duluth in June can be cool, and the Lake Superior scenery is pleasant.

There's also the party atmosphere before and after the races, making it an event for the townspeople as well as the visiting runners. The organizers probably spend as much money on entertainment as they do on appearance fees for elite athletes. And the recent addition of companion half-marathon and five-mile races doesn't seem to have subtracted from the main-event marathon.

first-time marathoners. In 1992, when Lorna Lyrek of Loretto, Minnesota, crossed the line at Grandma's, finishing with a time of 4:12:30, she became the 1,000th student of Bill Wenmark to finish a first marathon.

Wenmark, a former semipro ice hockey player and Vietnam veteran, has been instructing first-timers since 1981 in a program he runs for the American Lung Association in Minneapolis. He heads a club of marathoners called the American Lung Association Running Club (ALARC). Each spring and each summer, he accepts 45 hopeful marathoners into his classes: The spring group is preparing for Grandma's, and the summer group is aiming at Twin Cities. Since the program's inception, only five have failed to finish—and three of those later completed a marathon.

Lorna Lyrek was the 17th finisher among Wenmark's Beginning Marathon Class that spring. There had been active discussion about which class member would be the 17th to finish (and thus become the 1,000th Wenmark first-time marathoner). Not only was there a certain degree of celebrity attached to being number 1,000, but that person would also be awarded a plaque commemorating his or her achievement by the race organizers.

Bill Wenmark was born December 20, 1947, in Anoka, Minnesota. Ice hockey is an important sport in that part of the Midwest, and he excelled as a 215-pound defenseman on the rink in high school. His team sports career ceased after graduation from high school when he accepted a scholarship from the U.S. Navy to become a physician, attending the University of Maryland. He never did get a medical degree, but volunteered as a medical corpsman with the U.S. Marines and served in 1968 and 1969 in Vietnam.

Returning from the service in 1970, Wenmark focused his attention on health and fitness, and currently he owns two medical centers and two family practices. He is president and chief executive officer of NOW Care Medical Centers.

For recreation, he skated and jogged to keep in shape. In the fall of 1979, he decided it might be fun to run the City of Lakes Marathon that wound around several of the lakes in Minneapolis, a predecessor to the current Twin Cities Marathon. He finished on 23 miles of training. Not 23 miles a day. Not 23 miles a week. But 23 miles—total.

Wenmark finished the race in 5:57:37. "I died," he says. "I'm now in my second lifetime. The three days immediately following the race were three of the most miserable days I've had in my life. I paid the price. Every bone ached. Every muscle ached. Even my fingernails ached."

The City of Lakes Marathon followed a figure-eight course around Lakes Calhoun and Harriet; the final loop around Harriet was 2.8 miles. "That last loop, I was in nowhere land," says Wenmark. "I knew the finish line was at the top of the lake, and I had to circle it one more time, but I don't remember anything else. When I parked my car before the race, it had seemed close, but afterward, that was the longest walk in my life—yet it was a mere three blocks. When I got in to drive home, my legs were barely functioning. The car had a five-speed transmission, and I couldn't work the clutch pedal. I stayed in third gear all the way home."

Part of his problem was that he had trained for the marathon in a pair of Brand-X shoes that looked like they might have been purchased at a garage sale. For the race, however, he decided he needed decent footwear. Visiting a running store, he selected a popular model: gold with blue trim. The salesman suggested size 12; Wenmark, having recently won a prize in a weight-loss contest, didn't want to admit that his feet were that big. "I insisted on a half size smaller," he recalls. "After the marathon, I was lucky I still had toes.

"One of the reasons I'm so successful with first-time marathoners is that I made every mistake anyone ever made in preparing for my first 26-mile race," he says.

Turning Joggers into Runners

Nevertheless, Wenmark persisted in long distance running, which at the beginning of the 1980s was undergoing a transition from a cult sport enjoyed by a few to a mass sport embraced by growing numbers of once sedentary baby boomers. He was a volunteer member of the American Lung Association and in 1981, two years after his first marathon, convinced that organization to sponsor a class he would teach for first-time marathoners. "I had some medical training in exercise physiology, so I understood anatomy and what was going on inside the body. I thought, 'There's got to be a way to train for 26 miles and have fun.' " He developed a 13-week curriculum and contacted as guest lecturers well-known runners from the area—Garry Bjorklund, Dick Beardsley, Mike Slack, Barney and Jan Klecker, Alex Ratelle—and began teaching runners. His first class of 18 graduated at the 1981 City of Lakes Marathon.

Wenmark eventually chose 45 as the maximum number for his classes, although three times that number apply each spring or summer. He has enlisted 12 facilitators, experienced runners who work closely with individuals each class session. As the reputation of the class grew, the yellow ALARC shirts worn by class members in training became a status symbol. So too were the blue singlets they wore in their first marathon. Only after graduation and completion of their first marathon would class members be permitted to purchase the regular ALARC red singlet. "People come to us as joggers," says Wenmark, "and we turn them into runners."

He does this using a deceptively simple schedule. He explains: "Training involves a weekly long run, either Saturday or Sunday. Two days each week—Monday and Friday—are optional. They can be off days, or easy days if they like. If they do the long run on Saturday, they take Friday off. If Sunday, they rest Monday. I also encourage our class members to ride a stationary bike 15 to 30 minutes, five days a week. Wednesday is a moderate-distance run: to 13 miles, as the buildup proceeds. Tuesdays and Thursdays are anywhere from 6 to 8 miles. Also on Tuesday and Thursday, we look for terrain variation, rolling hills, and do fartlek late in the program."

The training program works. His experience in coaching 1,000 runners to cross the finish line—and cross it *comfortably*—has allowed Bill Wenmark to identify and break down what is needed for success in long distance running. He can point to 15 reasons for his success as a coach of first-time marathoners.

1. **Commitment.** Wenmark claims that within eight weeks after starting his class, the lifestyles of everybody in it will have changed: "Their social status will have changed, their nutrition will have changed, their relationship with their

family will have changed. They won't want to stay out late Saturday nights any more, because they have to do a long run the next morning." He believes that people must have the commitment to accept these major lifestyle changes. "You should run your first marathon for the right reasons," he says, "because you'll never be the same as a person again. You must want to do it, not do it because your boss did it or your spouse did it."

2. **Flexibility.** Wenmark dislikes the cookbook schedules often offered to runners. When interviewed for this book, he resisted providing a day-by-day schedule of how his runners train. He doesn't arbitrarily say that everybody must run 60 miles a week—or do speedwork on a certain day. He has trained first-timers of all ages from 18 to 72 (including his mother, who started running in 1985 and ran her fifth marathon in the 1992 Grandma's race at age 77). "Everybody's different," he says. "Some come with athletic backgrounds, some without. Obviously, there are different somatotypes [builds]. I don't want to clone them and say, 'You're all the same.' We establish different schedules for everybody. Some do 60 miles a week; some might do as little as 25."

3. **Support.** Wenmark subdivides his class, and volunteer facilitators work closely with a small number of beginners in a 1:5 ratio. (One advantage: Some women are more comfortable talking to other women about specifically female problems, such as, "What do I do if I have my period on marathon day?") He makes a point of focusing on the slowest members of the class. "We take care of the rear of the pack," he says. "I don't want anybody left alone on runs." ALARC is the largest running club in Minnesota, so support comes also from club members who shout encouragement when they see people wearing the familiar yellow shirts. "It's like graduating from college," says Wenmark. "You're known by the year of your graduation, and there's a common bond between those who came before and those who came after."

4. **Thoroughness.** "The most important thing about our program is that we don't miss one thing about what you need

to know to prepare for a marathon," says Wenmark. "We touch on psychological aspects and positive mental imaging. We provide nutrition assessment and physical therapy. We spend a lot of time teaching stretching and cross-training, so it's not just running. It's a holistic approach." He seeks to teach a lifestyle as much as how to finish a single marathon. After his students finish their first marathon, he wants them to continue as runners, embracing all the facets of the marathon lifestyle whether or not they run any more marathons.

5. **Praise.** Wenmark considers first-time marathoners a "rare commodity, because every experience is new." He says, "If they have never run 10 miles before in a single workout, achieving that goal becomes a cause for celebration. Then the 11th mile. Then the 12th. Each week brings a new achievement." And each new achievement receives praise.

6. **Respect.** Wenmark never runs his first-timers past 20 miles. "We never go the full distance," he says. "That's land for new exploration. In the race, they'll move into territory they've never visited before." He instills respect for the marathon, so that when his runners do venture beyond 20 the first time, the final 10-K is something special. "If they've behaved themselves to that point," he insists, "they will be successful."

7. **Practice.** The marathon, claims Wenmark, offers a classic example of success rewarded. "If you want to be successful in anything," he says, "it requires practice." One of his graduates is Harvey MacKay, author of the best-selling book, *Swim with the Sharks without Being Eaten Alive.* Wenmark has adopted one of MacKay's tenets: "Practice makes perfect. But perfect practice makes for success." Wenmark believes that by finishing a marathon, people can catch a glimpse of their own potential. They can then move on to be successful at other endeavors.

8. **Preparation.** "Do it the right way, which is the long way," says Wenmark. Shortcuts don't work. "The crowd watching the marathon will know it if you didn't prepare well enough," he says. "You'll either hurt big time or drop out."

He talks about people cramming for an exam not retaining the information as well as those who spread their study over a longer period of time. "You can't cram for a marathon," he says, "because the final exam for the marathon will never allow you to be successful if you take shortcuts."

9. **Groundwork.** Wenmark insists that his students accumulate a proper amount of base training before starting class. Nobody is accepted into the program unless they already are running at least 25 to 35 miles a week and have been training at that level at least five weeks. "You can't come in cold turkey," he warns. An interesting side point is that he sees more injuries (what he calls "nicks and dings") among those who sign up for the Grandma's class, which starts in March, rather than the Twin Cities class, which starts in July. He interprets that to mean that first-timers are likely to have not trained through the winter. The runners in the later marathon probably started training in the spring and have a few more months of base training. This additional base is what offers fall marathoners additional protection against injury.

10. **Simulation.** Wenmark simulates the marathon before the race. Anything that the students encounter during the 26.2 miles of the race, they will have encountered previously in practice at shorter distances. ALARC meets six days a week at three different sites, so there are ample opportunities to practice race strategies. Not only do class members run local, shorter races, they also do long runs planned to simulate marathon conditions, including aid stations with food and drink every two miles. One of the most popular events in the Twin Cities area is the ALARC 20-mile training run, two weeks before the marathon, with anywhere from 275 to 300 participants.

11. **Hydration.** Wenmark teaches his first-timers how to drink on the run, specifically how to *stop* running so they can drink more. Not only do they stop for what he calls "the pause that refreshes," but they follow a specific routine that includes stretching. "They stop a minimum of 19

times," he explains. "They take a drink. They stretch by bending forward. They drink again. They stretch by bending backwards. They drink. If any other body parts are tight, they stretch a third time." He guarantees that nobody who passes them by running through a water station will finish in front of them. He is rarely wrong. He also teaches them to eat (high-energy bars, Wheat Thins, saltine crackers), believing that if you're running five or six hours, fluids are not enough and you need to eat like an ultramarathoner.

12. **Proper weight.** Wenmark monitors weight closely, believing that—to a point—every pound of weight that his first-timers lose will make them faster. "Every pound you can get closer to your 'ideal body weight' is the equivalent of ten miles extra in your running diary," he says. For runners who are already lean, establishing that ideal weight is the secret and involves measurement of body fat percentages with calipers. Diet, combined with the extra miles run preparing for the marathon, helps runners approach their best weights. Wenmark stresses proper nutrition, beginning with the first class. He recommends trimming all visible fat from meat, claiming they can remove 70 percent of their fat calories by doing just that alone. He preaches the familiar dictum: "Eat breakfast like a king, lunch like a prince and dinner like a pauper." He believes that most people consume too many of their calories at the meals when they don't use the calories, quoting a study at the University of Minnesota, which found that a group fed a majority of their calories in the morning lost more weight than the same group fed the same amount in the evening.

13. **Cross-training.** Wenmark believes in cross-training and encourages his first-timers to practice other exercises. He suggests use of a stationary bicycle for 15 to 30 minutes, five days a week. His students do some weight lifting—light weights, high repetitions—for both upper- and lower-body development. "In running, you strengthen the back muscle groups but do little for the front of the body: the abdominals and the quads," he points out. Weight training

allows the balancing of these muscles and also provides the upper-body strength needed in the closing stages of the marathon. Push-ups, sit-ups and light work with dumbbells are important. "In the marathon, you hit the ground 37,000 times with your feet, but your arms are moving the same number of times, " he says. "So unless you also strengthen your arms, you're liable to fail."

14. **"Slow" work.** He avoids speedwork for beginners. "First-timers are learning how to run far, not how to run fast," he says. He emphasizes "time spent running," not how fast a certain distance is covered. Since finishing time is irrelevant, training methods to improve that time become unnecessary baggage.

Another reason Wenmark avoids speedwork is because he is trying to teach the body to burn fat by running slowly. And the slower the PR a runner sets, the easier it will be to better it in the next marathon.

15. **Attitude.** Wenmark considers attitude the most important word in the marathoner's lexicon. "It's an attitude about your new lifestyle," he says, "an awareness about the meaning of good health, a focus on the inevitable goal: the finish line, not the time on the clock when you cross that finish line."

And that is how you teach 1,000 runners to finish their first marathons.

CHAPTER 5

Striving to
IMPROVE

H ow do you improve as a marathoner? How do you run faster?
That's the key question for many runners. Getting to the finish
line of your first marathon is just a matter of preparation—as
coaches such as Bill Wenmark have proved time and time again.
Either through talent or a well-structured and progressive training program (or both), most people who set their minds upon
becoming marathoners succeed.

If they're hooked on the sport, their next goal is to get better.
They seek to run the fastest possible marathon they can in every
attempt, whether it's their 3rd or their 33rd time.

It's not that simple, but also not that difficult.

Tips from a Top Runner

Let's look at Doug Kurtis, the runner from Northville,
Michigan, who has run 131 marathons, about half of them sub-
2:20. Now into his forties, Kurtis probably has reached the point
of zero improvement. (He set his PR of 2:13:34 at the Mardi Gras
Marathon in New Orleans in 1982 on one of those perfect days
that every runner dreams of.) The principles Kurtis applies to
his training can apply to you as you attempt to narrow the gap
between your best time and his.

For the October 1991 issue of *Runner's World,* I wrote an article with Kurtis that was touted on the cover as: "26.2 Proven
Ways to Run a Better Marathon." This article apparently struck

a chord with many of our readers, judging from comments I heard afterward and letters the magazine received. Many of Kurtis's secrets are scattered throughout this book—along with the secrets of many other experienced runners—but four points in particular apply to the task faced by all of us as we seek to improve. Here, in Kurtis's words, are these four major points.

Consistency. The biggest key for me is that I'm built to run marathons: 5'7" and 130 pounds. But another factor is my consistency. My mileage remains the same week after week. There's no down time, no up time, no breaks. I could probably run 150 to 160 miles a week, but I would have a much harder time avoiding injuries. I recover well and rarely get injured. *When you're consistent with your training week after week, there's much less chance of entering a race undertrained or overtrained, both reasons why people get hurt or run poorly.* This is true for athletes in other sports as well.

Mileage. I have a strong incentive to do my twice-daily workouts and put in my 105 miles a week: High mileage permits me to run sub-2:20 marathons rather than run somewhat slower. Because of this, I win races and receive invitations to travel all over the world with expenses paid. For someone trying to run 3:20 or 4:20, the incentive might not be quite as high. *Everybody has a mileage level that's best for them.* Each person has to determine what's important to them and use that as a guide to dictate training level.

Intensity. A lot of people believe they have to train hard all the time. They feel they're not getting anything out of a workout unless they're running race pace. That's not true. *You can achieve a lot with slow workouts.* For me, a 7:00 pace is fast enough, and I often run slower. I'll sometimes start a workout running an 8:00 or 9:00 pace. When I'm training 105 miles a week, there's no way I can run hard every workout. Two things can happen: You can burn out if you run hard every day, or you can become injured.

Rest. *I'm not afraid to take days off.* Usually I average 15 to 20 rest days a year. I don't plan them in advance, but it's usually when something comes up: travel, or illness, or a family outing. It's good for me, and I probably should rest more often. One of the advantages of keeping your training consistent year-round is that when you do take a short rest, you lose very little of your training edge.

Let's consider Kurtis's four key points and the scientific principles behind them.

The Secrets of Improvement

Kurtis stresses *consistency.* If you're a beginning runner who has just finished your first marathon, you'll continue to improve if you do nothing but train consistently.

"When you're consistent with your training week after week," says Kurtis, "there's much less chance of entering a race undertrained or overtrained, both reasons why people get hurt or run poorly." Most established training programs for first-time marathoners last anywhere from three to nine months. Class leaders guide their students through a graduated schedule whose main feature is a long run that gets progressively longer (usually from 10 to 20 miles) as marathon day approaches. They send their students to the line usually undertrained and well rested, because experience has shown that to be the best way to ensure that they finish.

Better to be safe than sorry. And who can argue with success? Thus, most well-coached, first-time marathoners run their races without the training necessary to achieve peak performance, and run comfortably slower than their talents might allow. They finish thinking they probably could have run somewhat faster if they had trained harder.

They're right—they can. And so can you.

Steady Does It

Even without adopting a refined training schedule, most marathoners can improve merely by continuing to train at or near the same level. After three to nine months, you will have only begun to reap the benefits of that level of dedication. Your undertrained body will continue to improve, as long as you don't overtrain it. So keep running those long runs on the weekends, whether 20 miles or somewhat less. Keep running a medium run in the middle of the week. Take those one or two rest days weekly as suggested by Bill Wenmark in the previous chapter. Fill in the rest of the week with runs at various short distances and mix in some running at near your marathon pace. The accumulation of miles over a period of time will allow you to improve. You *will* get better.

The important thing is to maintain your fitness at a steady level. Research by John L. Ivy, Ph.D., at the University of Texas in Austin suggests that runners begin to detrain (lose their fitness) after 48 to 76 hours, and that it will take two days of *re*training to regain the fitness lost for every lost day of training. That doesn't mean you should never rest, but if you take long periods off, it will take you longer periods to come back.

That is why Doug Kurtis preaches consistency. You don't need to maintain continuous peak condition, but settle upon a consistent level of training that you know you can maintain for 12 months of the year. When it comes time to aim for a specific marathon, you can increase that level of training. The important goal is to maintain an effective endurance base.

The American College of Sports Medicine guidelines for fitness suggest three to four days of exercise a week, 20 to 60 minutes a day. That's the minimum fitness formula for maintaining good health, beyond which Kenneth H. Cooper, M.D., president and founder of the Cooper Aerobics Center in Dallas, Texas, suggests you're exercising for other reasons. For you, that will be true: Your reason is to stay in shape to run marathons. You'll need to—and want to—run more than the time alloted in Dr. Cooper's formula. But the basic pattern offered in the college's guidelines still apply to marathoners.

I coach the boys' and girls' cross-country teams at Elston High School in Michigan City and work with the distance runners there during the track season. Between seasons, I encourage my runners to keep diaries, and I try to examine those diaries periodically to monitor their conditioning programs. I discovered that the less dedicated ones would train hard for three or four days but then would miss three or four days of running. They thought they were staying in shape, but they were actually sliding backwards—as they proved when they appeared for practice the first day of the season. The ones who trained consistently improved; the others did not.

As a result, I told them: *Never go two days without running.* One day of missed training was no problem. That qualifies as rest. But two continuous days lost equalled lost conditioning— and inevitably meant poorer performances once the season began.

Finding Your Mileage Level

Doug Kurtis is a high-mileage trainer, and that's one of the secrets of his success. Most runners would crash if they attempted to mimic his 105 miles average per week, even after years of preparation, but Kurtis does not necessarily recommend that everybody train at his high level. He says, "Everybody has a mileage level that's best for them." Determining that level is tricky and may take several years of experimentation, but once you do, you can reap the benefits of success.

Norm Green, a Baptist minister from Wayne, Pennsylvania, who ran his first marathon at age 49—achieving an eventual (and amazing) PR of 2:25:51 at age 52—succeeded on 55 miles a week. During my years of peak performance, I found that I competed well in marathons on around 75 miles of weekly training. On those one or two occasions when I could edge my training mileage above 100 and hold it there for several months, I achieved peak performances. But I risked injury by doing so. And also boredom, because I found the twice-daily workouts necessary to achieve that mileage level robbed running of much of its joy.

Today, I find 40 weekly miles a more acceptable training level when I'm running 10-K races. When I'm aiming for a marathon, I try to push that level to 60 miles, with most of the extra mileage gained by adding one progressively longer run once a week. Think about it: All you need do to increase your weekly mileage from 40 to 60 is add a single workout of 20 miles.

The best way to determine your optimum mileage level is to keep a training diary. You can find various diaries at bookstores for recording your training, and there are even software programs that let you keep daily workout records in your computer. Or you can simply mark mileage on a wall calendar.

I record my workouts on special diary pages I keep in small, three-ring notebooks. There's a row of such notebooks on a shelf in my office, one for each year. I started the practice while Fred Wilt was coaching me in the 1960s (Fred is a 1948 and 1952 Olympian from Lafayette, Indiana, who later coached the women's teams at Purdue University). Each day, I recorded my workouts and related information. At the end of the week, I mailed Fred my diary pages for critiquing. Later, I designed a special diary format similar to his and had pages printed at a local printer for me and a few others to use.

My diary has spaces for the time of my run, location, temperature, surface, distance and what I did to warm up or cool down. There's also room for comments, as well as boxes to record pace-per-mile in races or interval quarters run in workouts. It sounds complicated, but it actually takes a minute each day. Then when things go wrong—or right—I can examine my training and determine the reasons.

During special periods of time—such as when I'm preparing for a marathon or peaking for maximum performance at the World Veterans Championships—I take poster board and a black marker and make my own diary calendars showing three, six or nine months, whatever the training for that particular race requires. I'll tack the poster-sized calendar to a cork wall in my basement that I pass each day before and after running. It serves as both a visual record of what I have done and a reminder of what I have to do. In addition to what I write in my diary, I'll mark weekly mileages and sometimes specific key workouts, such as the distance of my long run.

I use it as motivation, but also as a safety net. If I notice that I have run four consecutive weeks at the 50-mile-plus level (which is high for me), I may think, "Hmmmm. Maybe I should back off my training for a week to avoid getting injured."

Finding the appropriate training level is not easy—particularly because that level may change as you get stronger or get older—but it is essential if you want to improve as a marathoner.

Slowing It Down

If there's one difference between fast runners and those who finish back in the pack, it's that the fast runners seem to have no qualms about running slowly. They're not embarrassed about it. Doug Kurtis says, "You can achieve a lot with slow workouts." He's quite happy to train at a 7:00 pace, nearly two minutes a mile slower than his race pace in marathons, and he sometimes starts workouts running an 8:00 or 9:00 pace.

I feel the same way as Kurtis, although at this point in my career, I run much slower than that. In fact, I'll do some workouts at a 10:00 pace, or slower. If you station yourself near my house with a spyglass, you may even catch me cruising in at the end of a long run at 12:00 a mile. That's a broad gap from the near 6:00 pace I might run in a 10-K, or the 7:00 pace in a marathon, but my goal is to perform well in important races, not in every daily workout.

The important message in Kurtis's comment is not that he trains slowly, but that he trains *differently* each day. If I had to cite one mistake made by inexperienced marathoners when they seek to improve their performances, it is that they run too many of their miles at the same pace, and over the same distance. There's little variety, and that limits their improvement.

If I'm running slowly on one day, it's probably because I ran hard the day before—or want to run hard the day after. To improve, you need to add intensity to your program. You may not necessarily need to run sprints on the track, but you need to at least run as fast as race pace. Very few runners can run race pace day after day. Norm Green is one of those rare runners: At his peak, he averaged faster than 6:00 miles in training. Most runners, however, would break if they attempted to duplicate that feat—which Norm is first to admit. In order to train at a high level of intensity on certain days, most of us need to train at a low level of intensity on other days. That's where slow running comes in.

Scientifically Speaking

From a scientific standpoint, slow running is important for several reasons.

Caloric burn. It varies from runner to runner, depending on size and metabolism, but most of us burn 100 calories for every mile we run. Burn 3,600 calories by running 36 miles and you lose one pound. But it doesn't matter how fast you run those miles. You can even walk and burn the same number of calories per mile. Calorie loss is related to foot-pounds: the amount of effort (i.e., energy) it takes to push a body of a specific weight forward. You can run a 5:00 mile or a 10:00 mile, and you'll still burn 100 calories for covering the identical distance.

One means of attaining maximum performance is to achieve optimum body weight and optimum body fat percentage. You can do that just as easily with long, steady distance: It will take you somewhat longer than if you ran those miles fast, but you're less likely to become injured.

Sparing glycogen. Exercise physiologists also say that when you run slowly, your body has time to metabolize fat as a source of energy. When you run fast your body burns glycogen, a derivative of carbohydrate, as its preferred energy source. Glycogen is stored in the muscle and is a more efficient fuel in the sense that the body can metabolize it more rapidly than fat. But by training slowly, you apparently teach your muscles to become more efficient at also metabolizing fat, thus sparing glycogen stores for those last few miles in the marathon.

No Running

With that idea in mind, realize that *no* running is as important a part of the marathoner's training guide as *slow* running. Kurtis, who averages 15 to 20 rest days a year, says he's not afraid to take days off. That amounts to 1 or 2 days off a month—which isn't much—but some runners don't even rest that much. In *Lore of Running,* Timothy Noakes, M.D., analyzes the training patterns of several dozen expert runners. He looks at reasons they failed and reasons they succeeded. In the former case, often it was because they trained too hard and were too unwilling to take days off.

A prime example is Ron Hill, a British marathoner with a 2:09:28 best, whom Dr. Noakes suspected was as much interested in keeping his streak of double workouts unbroken as he was in winning the 1972 Olympic marathon. An earlier British runner, Jim Peters, trained relentlessly, day after day, almost without pause, once running a half dozen miles at a 5:00 pace the day before setting one of his world records. Yet in two of his most important races (the 1952 Olympics and 1954 Commonwealth Games), Peters failed to finish. At the Commonwealth Games in British Columbia on a hot day, he collapsed while leading and within sight of the marathon finish line. He retired after that race out of fear that his intense will might cause him to seriously hurt himself. Dr. Noakes suggests that had he alternated hard and easy training days and tapered for his races—common practices among marathoners today—Peters might have run even faster.

Knowing when to back off and take a complete day off—or even more—is one of the secrets of marathon success. It is not easy, since the traditional work ethic that has made many people successes suggests that more is better. That training calendar on my basement wall would be more of a hindrance than a help if it pushed me to run extra miles just to achieve mileage levels I may have planned months ago—without considering whether I have a cold, or failed to get enough sleep the night before, or am overly fatigued because of having spent most of the previous day on an airplane.

Rest is essential to success. Bill Wenmark programs two days of rest into each week for his first-time marathoners. Most people reading this book understand that tapering before a marathon—cutting training mileage the last week or two before the race—is important to ensuring success.

Less recognized is the necessity for rest and mini-tapers all through the marathon training program. Take a day off; it won't hurt.

Does this message contradict the earlier one related to consistency, the importance of maintaining a steady schedule? Not at all, because who can better afford to take days off than someone who trains consistently?

If you hope to get better as a marathon runner, you need to pay attention to the basic elements championed by Doug Kurtis—consistency, mileage, intensity and rest—but those are only four of the routes available to you. Let's consider next the benefits of the long run.

CHAPTER 6

Building Up
YOUR
MILEAGE

Just about any marathon coach will agree that building up your weekly mileage is essential for success in any long-distance event. "You need time on your legs," says Susan Kinsey, a coach from La Mesa, California.

But how much time? Atlanta's Jeff Galloway, a former high-mileage Olympian, has made a very successful career of teaching runners to finish their first marathons on the least amount of mileage possible. Three or four days a week training coupled with some long runs is all you need, says Galloway. And it works: More than 98 percent of those in Galloway's marathon program finish their first marathon, some on as little as 20 to 30 weekly miles.

The coaches surveyed for this book agreed that about 35 miles a week was adequate to finish a marathon, 55 miles to finish well. Most elite runners believe 100-plus-mile weeks are necessary to excel, but research suggests anything more than 75 miles a week is a waste.

How many miles do you need to run each week? It depends on your goals, your abilities and your schedule—and in some cases, whom you listen to.

What the 100-Milers Have to Say

Before the 1980 Olympic marathon trials, a survey of the American contenders showed that nearly all of them trained more than 100 miles a week—somewhat disheartening for the aspiring marathoner now doing 30 miles a week and hoping to work up to 50 or 60.

Bill Rodgers and Frank Shorter, 1976 Olympians and two of the most successful and consistent American road racers at that time, trained 140 miles a week. "I always felt best when doing high mileage," says Rodgers. Alberto Salazar ran 130 miles a week before the 1984 marathon trials. Carlos Lopes, 1984 Olympic champion, ran 140 on average. Joan Benoit Samuelson, the women's gold medalist in the 1984 Games, also ran over 100. Ingrid Kristiansen ran as far as 125 miles weekly prior to breaking Samuelson's world record in the 1985 London Marathon. A survey of the current crop of elite marathoners probably would reveal similar mileage totals.

Tom Fleming, a 2:12:05 marathoner with several second-place finishes at Boston, claims such high mileage is necessary for excellence. "You have to do 140 miles a week to get into the 2:12 bracket," he says. "And you have to maintain that mileage. Most people can't do it. Anyone can run 140 for three or four weeks, but that's not enough. I'd love to be able to have ten months of 140-mile weeks." Bill Rodgers, he points out, ran at that level during his best three years: "His body held up under the stress of the hard training, and the result was that he was the best marathoner in the world."

You Can Excel on Less

Not all top distance runners think you need this many miles, however. Don Kardong of Spokane, Washington, finished fourth in the 1976 Olympic marathon (2:11:16) with less mileage than most top marathoners, averaging 80 to 90 miles most weeks. "My feeling is that people pick 100 because it's a nice, round number," he says. "But 88 is an even *rounder* number."

Consider Benji Durden, a top masters runner from Boulder, Colorado, and coach of top female marathoner Kim Jones. When he ran 110 miles a week at an average pace of 6:30 per mile,

Durden had PRs of 29:21 for the 10-K and 2:10:41 for the marathon, and made the 1980 Olympic marathon team.

But Durden found the stress imposed by that much training too intense. In 1983, he cut his mileage to a still-imposing 85 to 95 miles a week—and set new PRs. He improved to 28:37 for the 10-K and 2:09:58 for the marathon, third at Boston. "I believe you can be a successful performer on low mileage, as little as 70 to 80 miles a week," Durden now claims. Granted, most of us wouldn't consider 70 to 80 miles a week low mileage, but it is for an elite runner.

Craig Virgin, a three-time Olympian and two-time world cross-country champion, was another relatively low-mileage runner. While setting PRs of 27:29.2 for 10,000 meters and 2:10:26 for the marathon (in a second-place finish at Boston in 1981), Virgin averaged 90 to 95 miles a week. He didn't run his first 100-mile week until his junior year in college and, except when training for his infrequent marathons, rarely strung 100-mile weeks together.

"I don't think they give any awards for workouts," said Virgin, who's now retired. "To the best of my knowledge, there are no gold medals for 'Most Mileage.' If it was the end of the week, and I had 98 miles in, I didn't go for a third workout that day to get 100. That won't make the difference between winning and losing. It's what you do with that 100 miles a week, and I think people forget about that."

What Those Miles Accomplish

The late physiologist Al Claremont claimed that high mileage helps you better utilize glycogen, the starchlike substance stored in the liver and muscles and changed into a simple sugar as the body needs it. Carbohydrates in our diet are our main source of glycogen, one reason spaghetti is such a popular prerace meal for marathoners. Glycogen is the preferred fuel for running, but your levels can become depleted within 60 to 90 minutes. Thereafter, your source of fuel is fat, which is metabolized less efficiently.

Claremont believed high-mileage running in essence teaches your body to burn more fat along with the glycogen, stretching the duration of your reserves from 60 to 90 minutes to two hours or more. He explained: "Top marathoners are probably so efficient in metabolizing both fats and glycogen throughout the length of their race because of the vast volume of their training that they probably rarely deplete their stores. As a result, they don't hit the Wall."

William J. Fink, of Ball State University in Muncie, Indiana, suggests that volume training may result in a more efficient use of your muscle fibers. "When a runner doubles his training mileage, we often see no change in his maximum oxygen uptake, the ability to deliver oxygen to the muscles," explains Fink. This, he says, indicates that something else—perhaps improved muscle fibers—causes the better performances.

Jack H. Wilmore, Ph.D., at the University of Texas at El Paso, suggests there is a psychological effect to high mileage as well. "When you do 100 miles a week, your legs are chronically fatigued," he comments. "Then when you finally do taper before an important race, it makes you feel all the stronger. The same would hold true for a 30-mile-a-week runner who, through a gradual buildup, achieved an ability to train comfortably at 60."

Finally, Dr. Wilmore says mileage helps your body adapt to the punishment that occurs during marathons—in ways that scientists can't yet explain. "When I'm out of shape and I race at long distances, everything hurts," he says. "It feels like my connective tissues are coming apart. But when I'm ready for a marathon and have put in the miles, everything moves smoothly."

The Point of Diminishing Returns

Research from exercise laboratories, however, suggests that many of the long miles done by runners in the past may have been wasted—and in fact may have contributed to chronic overtraining that resulted in poorer, rather than better, performances. "You may run far," says David Martin, Ph.D., a U.S. Olympic team consultant, "but you don't run far long."

David L. Costill, Ph.D., director of the Human Performance Laboratory at Ball State, has measured beginning, average and elite runners, as well as athletes in other sports. He believes that there exists a finite limit beyond which athletes cease to improve. For runners, he suspects the limit is 50 to 75 weekly miles. "The amount of physiological improvement beyond that is almost insignificant," says Dr. Costill.

In one case documented in Dr. Costill's book, *Inside Running,* his lab studied two marathoners who resumed training after six-month layoffs due to injuries. Dr. Costill supervised muscle biop-

The Long Run

It has become a weekend tradition for so many American runners: the long run. If you call the homes of most distance runners on a Sunday at 7:00 A.M., you'll find they're either already out running or just about to head out the door.

Running far is not only enjoyable, but also essential to success in distances from 10-K to the marathon. "The single long run is as important as high mileage in a marathoner's training program," claims Alfred F. Morris, Ph.D., director of health and fitness at the National Defense University in Washington, D.C. Tom Grogon, a coach from Cincinnati, Ohio, ranks it second only to "raw talent."

Robert Wallace, a 2:13 marathoner who placed ninth at Boston in 1982 and is a part-time coach in Dallas, says: "I still love those long, easy runs on Sunday. They're the mainstay of any training program. You don't get results immediately. It's like saving pennies: Put them in a jar and over a year you accumulate $50 to $60."

Wallace favors slow workouts rather than fast for the long runs. "High-quality [fast] runs are too hard on a weekly basis," he says. "Run low-quality and you can get out every weekend. I like to see 10-K runners go 14 to 16 miles; marathoners go 20 to 22 miles, several minutes slower than race pace."

Joe Friel, coach and founder of a running store called Foot of the Rockies in Fort Collins, Colorado, considers it essential to build an endurance base. He has his runners do at least one long run every week, or every other week. "Every ten

sies and treadmill tests for VO_2 max as the pair gradually increased their weekly mileages.

Dr. Costill wrote: "As one might have predicted, the muscles showed dramatic improvements in aerobic capacity with as little as 25 miles of running per week. [Their] max values increased when they increased their weekly mileages to 50 and then 75

days would be perfect," says Friel, "but that's tough to fit into a work schedule."

David Cowein, an ultramarathoner from Morrilton, Arkansas, runs long once a month for two to six hours. "I'll usually run trails," he says. "If I did a run that long on roads, I'd be sore the next day, but trails are easier on my body. I'll run far, but I'll also run slowly, walking up hills if necessary."

Runners often do their long run in groups. "It's great to run with a group, because it can be lonely out there," says Wallace, who has a Sunday group of 20 that starts from a racquetball club in Flower Mound, a suburb of Dallas. "Even when I ran fast times, I always trained with the 3:00 and 3:30 runners," he says. "I just wanted to run long and didn't care at what pace."

Although I usually prefer running my longest runs solo (because I can slow down as much as I want if I start feeling tired), I frequently join members of the Dunes Running Club each Sunday morning at 8:00 at a parking lot near Lake Michigan on Kemil Road east of the Indiana Dunes State Park, about an hour's drive from Chicago. We'll run anywhere from 60 minutes to several hours on trails that wind up and down sand dunes and along a ridge with marvelous views of the lake or the inland marshes. Such runs can condition the mind as much as the body. (If you're ever in the area, join us.)

So don't call a long-distance runner early on a Sunday morning. If you don't get a sleepy spouse, you'll most likely get an answering machine.

miles per week. Beyond that level of training, however, our laboratory tests found no additional gains in endurance. During a one-month period they even trained at 225 miles per week, with no improvement in endurance."

In tests of other athletes, Dr. Costill was unable to detect any differences in oxygen uptake scores between runners who ran 60 miles weekly and those doing twice that mileage. "There may be some psychological reasons for running high mileage," he concedes, "but we haven't been able to measure it."

When working with swimmers, Dr. Costill found that they *improved* when their mileage was cut. When Ball State swimmers cut their daily mileage from 10,000 yards to 5,000 yards, everyone on the squad set new PRs—some by significant margins.

Fitting the Miles In

So what does all this mean to those of us who dream only of qualifying for Boston or setting a new PR? "There's no mystery about how you improve your endurance," says Lee Fidler, a running coach from Stone Mountain, Georgia, with a marathon PR of 2:15:03. "You just increase volume. I ran 110 miles a week ten years in a row, but not everybody can do that. For most people, 60 is plenty."

While you can finish a marathon on only 30 miles a week, to finish well you need to push your mileage up to the 55- or 60-mile-a-week level. To do so, you should make a gradual progression in increments of 10 percent a week, says Fidler. Every third or fourth week, drop back close to the starting point to recover. Fidler says: "If you build constantly week after week, you get stronger, but you also find your break point. It's best to approach your break point without reaching it. You advance in steps. Go up two or three steps, drop back one or two steps, then hop back to where you were and start stepping again."

Joe Catalano of East Walpole, Massachusetts, has coached everyone from beginning joggers to his former wife, Patti Lyons Catalano, who had a marathon best of 2:27:51. He believes people vary in their ability to increase mileage: He recommends a gradual climb, adding five extra miles a week for a top runner but fewer for others. "The endurance base is the single most important factor in getting fit," he advises. "People worry about speed, but if you concentrate first on mileage and improving your strength, you can move to the speed phase later."

Thom Hunt, a distance runner from San Diego, California, whose best marathon time is 2:12:14, often varies his mileage from week to week and from season to season. He usually runs between 85 and 105 miles a week, slightly higher immediately before marathons. But he varies his workouts. "I might run 105 one week, 115 the week after that, then go down and run a 90," says Hunt. "Rest is an important part of a training program. There are times of the year when you just go to the beach."

The Perils of the Numbers Game

What you need to beware of is concentrating on how many miles you're running to the exclusion of everything else. Many runners become fixated on high mileage, feeling that if they fail to reach their weekly mileage goal they remain unfulfilled. They begin worrying by Wednesday or Thursday: "Am I going to make it this week?" At this point, they're running more for their diaries than themselves. They're also spending a lot of time running "junk miles"—miles that have no effect on fitness or performance.

While high mileage may help produce better times, simply *adding* mileage may not guarantee success either for the world-class athlete or the dedicated jogger who dreams of Boston. Quality must be mixed with quantity to produce maximum results. Don Kardong says: "People are too conscious of high mileage and not conscious enough about quality. It's a natural outcome of keeping a running diary. You become very concerned with how many miles you ran this week, but not with how fast you ran them. In the next few years we may see a shift back to quality rather than quantity."

Dr. Martin believes that much of the so-called rehabilitative running that elite runners do between hard runs may simply deaden their legs. "One of the secrets to remaining fresh," he says, "is to limit impact time, the number of times your feet strike the pavement."

Some runners jump from 50 to 75 miles to the "magic" 100 by

simply adding a second workout to their day. Dr. Martin has his doubts about the gains from multiple workouts. "Run 5 miles each morning, and multiply that by seven, and you get 35 miles," he says. "If you add that to 65 miles of hard training in the afternoon, you can write 100 in your training diary. But does that make you a better runner?"

Getting the Most from Your Mileage

And if you're trying to beef up your training, you may find it difficult to find time to get the miles in. You may be able to work out twice a day if your profession is running, but if you have other interests—a job, a family or other demands or pursuits—trying to cram a second workout into a busy schedule may not be worth it. You can, however, maximize the benefits you get from your single workout.

Dr. Martin compares two hypothetical runners. One trains 15 miles a day by running 7 in the morning and 8 in the evening. The other trains 10 daily with a single run. "Figure that it's going to take 3 miles to warm up and another mile to cool down. So where's the hard training?" he asks.

The hard training comes in the middle of a workout. The first runner in his morning workout runs 3 warm-up miles, pushes 3 hard, then uses 1 to cool down. His second workout is 3 warm-up miles, 4 hard miles, and 1 cool-down mile. In 15 miles of training the first runner has run hard only 7 miles.

Meanwhile, Dr. Martin's other runner may run only 10 miles, but 6 of them are hard. In addition to cutting running time, he also has eliminated the need for dressing and undressing and taking a shower one more time.

"Nowadays, with runners holding jobs and doing promotional work," says Dr. Martin, "they have more to do than just sit around all day and dream about running. One ten-mile run gives them more productive time for their other activities, and the end result is better fitness."

Also fewer injuries. Increasing your mileage is like throwing a pass in football: Three things can happen, two of them bad. In football, the options are complete, incomplete or intercepted. In running, you may set a PR, run poorly from fatigue or become injured. Most running injuries result from training mistakes, says orthopedist Stan James, M.D. "Often, they're due to high mileage."

Invariably, those who continue to run well into their forties and beyond are those who minimize the destructive effects of high mileage and maximize the efficiency of the miles they do.

Finding the Mileage That's Right for You

Top marathoners talk about "red-lining," a term borrowed from auto racers. The red line is the mark on the tachometer that marks the safety zone: If you consistently rev your engine higher, it disintegrates.

In running, red-lining means pushing your training to achieve maximum efficiency and your best performances. But if you push past your red line, you risk injury or breakdown.

A beginning runner might red-line after a gradual buildup at 30 miles. Or 45. Or 60. There are physiological limits: Too many miles too soon result in injuries such as strained tendons and ligaments, stress fractures, chronically dead legs and a persistent feeling of fatigue.

There are also psychological limits. Some runners can't cope with dressing, running and showering all the time—plus deal with the need for extra rest. Not only does 100 miles weekly require ten or more hours of actual running time, it requires a lot of recuperative time. One of the coaches in our survey suggested that elite runners need three to four hours of rest daily *plus* seven to eight hours of sleep each night.

Nobody can define the precise point between undertraining and overtraining, the point where optimum benefits occur. And this point certainly differs for different athletes. While one runner might thrive on 60 miles a week, another might need 90 and a third might need 120 to excel. It's also possible that this level may change at different points in an athlete's career.

In general, the runner who can increase training mileage should expect to improve as long as quality is not sacrificed for quantity. The key is to increase mileage gradually and to pay careful attention to how your body reacts.

CHAPTER 7

SPEEDWORK
for Distance Runners

D ark clouds hovered on the horizon as I drove eastward late on a spring afternoon toward Eagle Lake. The temperature was in the 60s, but dropping. Thunderstorms had rattled sporadically through the area during the past few hours. Only a few drops of rain had hit my windshield, but I found out later that others in the class had driven through heavy rain.

It was a Thursday in mid-April as we continued to prepare for the Sunburst Marathon in June. That evening, class members were scheduled to run 16 miles in their progression to a maximum long run of 20 before tapering to marathon day. But I didn't want to run that far, or that hard. I already had done my long run earlier in the week, so I decided to cut that night's distance to 11 and do some speedwork.

We were to run a preprepared course circling Eagle Lake on which my co-leader, Ron Gunn, had chalked mile marks so we knew how far we had to go. While driving toward Eagle Lake, I had decided to slice 5 miles from the planned workout and start at the 11-to-go mark. (Gunn drives class members to different starting points, depending on how far they want to run.)

I started slowly, as part of a planned warm-up. I ran the first two miles at an 8:30 pace, allowing several class members to move out ahead of me. I weighed how I felt: decent, but fatigued and a bit stiff from my long run earlier in the week. I would be running a 15-K in Kalamazoo, Michigan, on Saturday. It made sense to cruise comfortably and save energy for that race, the last formal test of my conditioning before the marathon.

But at the 9-to-go mark, I started to push hard. I shifted gear into what Jack Daniels, Ph.D., once called "cruise control." This is fast (but controlled) running, a phrase familiar to most serious runners.

I swept past several class members and continued at that pace until I crossed an "8" on the road. I punched my watch: 6:09 for the mile. I floated through the next mile, taking nearly ten minutes, then spurted again. Twice more I did the same at a nearly equal pace. Finally, I finished with two slow miles, coming in with a pair of runners I caught who had started at a different point along the course.

Later, I recorded that workout in my diary as 4 × 1 mile (one-mile jog between) with a two-mile warmup and a two-mile cooldown, a classic speed workout featuring repeats.

Who Needs Speedwork?

Speedwork! That's a scary word, a frightening concept to a lot of marathoners, who reason that there's nothing speedy about the pace at which they run 26-mile races. If so, why do speedwork, with its ultimate threat of injury? Most marathoners want to run *far,* not run fast. One runner who picked up a copy of *Run Fast* at an expo where I was selling copies grunted, "I don't want to run fast."

Fair enough. If you're a marathoner, you probably only need do speedwork if you want to improve your performances.

Does that grab your attention?

Speedwork is an effective way to train, even though its application that evening ruined my race in Kalamazoo on the weekend. With sore muscles, I failed to run any one mile as fast as I had that Thursday in practice. Bad judgment on my part? Perhaps, but I rationalized that my goals were long range: the marathon later that spring and still other races beyond. But in all honesty, I had operated on instinct when I chose to run fast, because it was a good night for running.

That's not a bad reason, but the more pressing reason to include speedwork in your training program—even for marathons—is to improve performance. "Speedwork coupled with overdistance can bring a runner to any goal," states Paul Goss, a coach and duathlete from Foster City, California. According to Alfred F. Morris, Ph.D., with the National Defense University in Washington, D.C., "It is important for runners to learn to run fast, so that the marathon pace feels comfortable." Adds Frank X. Mari, a coach from Toms River, New Jersey: "You will never see full potential as a marathon runner until you develop your full potential as a sprinter." Coach Keith Woodard of Portland, Oregon, adds: "You have to be able to run fast at short distances before you can run fast at long distances."

First-time marathoners, as mentioned in chapters 2 and 3, need give little attention to speedwork: Their main goal is to gradually (but gently) increase their mileage to permit them to finish a 26-mile race. Improving marathoners probably should also focus their attention on determining what level of high-mileage training (explained in chapters 4, 5 and 6) works best for them. But after you've been running for several years and you begin to shave seconds off your PRs instead of minutes, or if you start to slip backward, it's time to turn to speedwork. In the chapter on "Interval Training" in *Run Fast,* I quoted University of Oregon track coach Bill Dellinger as identifying that form of speedwork as "[developing] speed in a runner more quickly than any other form of training."

Well said, and most experienced marathoners know the value of speedwork, whether or not they practice it regularly. "Speed is my weakness, and I need to work on it," concedes Julie Isphording-Boaz, a 1984 Olympic marathoner. One time when I was visiting Cincinnati on business, I met her and a friend at 5:30 A.M. downtown near my hotel, and we ran across the Ohio River into Covington, Kentucky, to a high school track. The three of us had to climb a fence to get in, and it was still dark, but Isphording-Boaz ran 8 × 800 meters, jogging 400 between. Soon after, she won the Los Angeles Marathon. (Another favorite workout of hers is 5 × 1600 meters, also jogging 400 between.)

How You Benefit

Although long-distance runners concede that speedwork forms an integral part of any well-designed training regimen, not every marathoner uses it as part of his or her training. One reason is unfamiliarity. Many of today's adult runners didn't compete in track or on cross-country teams in high school, and speedwork and running tracks feel foreign to them.

There is also an element of fear, both of the unknown and of injury—with some justice, as training at a high intensity can cause you to hurt yourself. It also can *hurt,* and the burning sensation you get in your lungs and the ache in your legs seem more threatening than the less piercing fatigue you encounter on the roads. Usually after a hard workout on the track, particularly early in the season, my legs are sore for several days.

Also, you can't carry on a decent conversation while doing speedwork. When I did those early-morning interval halves at the Covington track with Julie Isphording-Boaz and her friend, I was hanging on for dear life. Only later, jogging back across the river into downtown Cincinnati, could we resume our conversation.

Nevertheless, there are ten good reasons why every long distance runner should do speedwork on a track.

1. **Performance.** This is the most valid reason. You will run faster. That's guaranteed. Numerous laboratory studies prove that adding speed training to an endurance base can take seconds off your 10-K times and minutes off your marathon bests. And runner after runner will testify to the value of including regular speed sessions in their long-distance program. Melvin H. Williams, Ph.D., director of the Human Performance Laboratory at Old Dominion University in Norfolk, Virginia, only began training seriously in his midthirties. After a half dozen years of mainly long-distance training, his performance times stalled in the 2:50s for the marathon. After he cut mileage and added speedwork, he dropped his PR to 2:33:30 at age 44. "By training faster," says Dr. Williams, "you improve specific muscles used at higher speeds. You also improve your anaerobic threshold, which allows you to run a faster pace and remain aerobic. If you can run faster at short distances, you can increase your absolute ability at longer distances, too."

2. **Form.** One of the best ways I know—in fact, the *only* way—to improve form is by running fast in practice. If you

can learn to run more efficiently (exercise physiologists prefer the term *economically*), you will perform better at all distances and levels. I'm not sure why speed training improves your running form. Maybe you recruit different muscles. Maybe you force yourself to move more smoothly. Maybe by learning how to run at speeds faster than race pace, you're more relaxed when you do run that pace in a marathon. Maybe it's all of those reasons. Whatever the reason, it works.

3. **Variety.** Running the same course and the same distance at the same pace day after day can become tedious. To keep running exciting, you need variety. "Keeping workouts varied is one way to ensure success," says coach Joe Catalano, from East Walpole, Massachusetts. Catalano has his runners do speedwork on the roads, on trails and on the track. Many roadrunning clubs organize speed workouts as a benefit to their members.

4. **Excitement.** Running alone through scenic trails provides its own pleasure, but tracks can have a level of activity that can stimulate you in your workouts. "Usually I prefer to do my fast running at a track where something is going on, even if it's only soccer practice and nobody's watching me," says Doug Kurtis, the runner from Northville, Michigan, who has run 131 marathons. "It's often hard to run when nobody's around."

   I used to train frequently at Stagg Field on the campus of the University of Chicago. There always seemed to be a half dozen activities going on simultaneously: rugby in the infield, tennis behind the stands, several softball games on an adjoining field, kids playing in the sand of the long jump pit, people doing yoga and track athletes practicing multiple events. There was an electricity about being in the middle of this whirlwind of athletic activity that I found enormously appealing.

5. **Convenience.** "There are tracks in every city and town," says Catalano, "so it's very convenient to find one to do your workouts." Another important point: You can obtain maximum benefit in minimum time by doing speedwork.

"My clients don't have much time," notes Robert Eslick, a coach of adult runners from Nashville, Tennessee, "so short workouts appeal to them."

Here's a workout taught to me by Fred Wilt, one of my former coaches. Head to the track and run eight laps, which is two miles (3200 meters). Run the first four laps (1600 meters) at a comfortable warmup pace. Then, without stopping, run the next 200 meters hard, the following 200 easy, and repeat for a total of four more laps. You're done, and your workout will have taken less than 20 minutes. That's an interval workout that would be expressed as 4 × 200 (200 jog). The final 200 jog serves as your cooldown, and then you're in the car heading home for dinner. (The same workout—once you learn the pattern—can be done on the road or on trails as well as on a track.)

6. **Concentration.** One of the skills that separates the good runners from the almost-good runners is an ability to focus their attention for the entire period of the race, whether it's a mile or a marathon. Dissociating is a good strategy for beginning marathoners, but not for people who want to run fast. When your mind wanders during a marathon, you inevitably slow down. If you stay focused, you learn how to concentrate all body systems to sustain a steady pace, conserve your energy and maintain your running form. Eslick suggests that repeats between ¾ mile and 1½ miles simulate the concentration and pacing feel needed in a marathon. It takes *total* concentration to run fast on a track; once you master this skill, you can transfer it to your road runs.

7. **Safety.** You can't get hit by a car while running on a track, and you probably won't be chased by a dog either. If you're in the company of others, it reduces the danger of being mugged. On a hot or cold day, if you become overheated or overchilled or overfatigued, you can just walk off the track and head for your car or the locker room: You don't have to worry about being caught three miles from home and trudging those final miles at a diminishing pace. Also, there are usually drinking fountains at running tracks, and toilets nearby.

8. **Companionship.** Willie Sutton once was asked why he robbed banks, and his response was, "Because that's where the money is." Well, tracks are where the runners are. On a track you can seek company and training partners, which are important if you want to push yourself. It sometimes becomes difficult to motivate yourself to train hard alone. With someone running those interval quarters with you, you can get a better workout and improve. But beware: A companion danger is that you can train *too* hard, resulting in staleness or injury. On balance, however, your running will improve if you find running partners with whom you enjoy training.

9. **Motivation.** Your running also will improve if you can find a coach to guide you in your training. A second variation of the Willie Sutton rule is that you find coaches at tracks. Because it's difficult to watch runners and monitor their strengths and weaknesses when they are scattered all over a road, most coaches prefer to gather people in groups for speedwork sessions. Probably the single most important asset a coach can offer any runner is motivation. Any runner can select one of the many training programs offered in this and other books, but only a skilled coach can motivate you and guide you to follow that program properly.

10. **Pleasure.** Just as it feels good for a tennis player to stroke the ball perfectly over the net or for a golfer to loft a well-aimed shot to the green, it also feels good to run fast. There's a certain tactile pleasure in doing any activity well, an experience that in running I call "feeling the wind in your hair." One way to achieve the pleasure of fast running is to run short distances interspersed with adequate periods of rest. In other words, speedwork. And because speedwork inevitably will allow you to improve your performance on race day, that will add to your pleasure, too.

Varieties of Speed

I defined speedwork in *Run Fast* as "any training done at race pace or faster." In that book I was offering advice for runners seeking to improve their 5-K and 10-K times, so I related race pace to how fast they ran those distances. If you run the marathon in 3:30, you run at an approximate pace of 8:00 per mile, but to go out and run a half dozen miles at your marathon pace—which most experienced runners could achieve easily— would not constitute speedwork. Speedwork for marathoners is training done at a pace significantly faster than you would run in a marathon. Your 10-K pace still remains an excellent benchmark.

To further define speedwork, I probably should add that it usually involves *bursts* of fast running (at race pace) followed by periods of slower running, or rest. That's essential, because most runners probably can only achieve race pace for long distances when well motivated and rested—in other words, in the race itself. To achieve race pace in practice, they need to cut their race distance in segments, and rest between those segments. If you were a competitor at 5000 meters, you could run 12 × 400 meters in a workout, resting short periods after each 400, and simulate some of the stress of your race as well as practicing race pace. A marathon runner wouldn't do 26 × 1 mile in a single workout, but the principle is the same.

There are different ways to do speedwork. Some ways work better for marathoners than for runners competing at shorter distances. You can run repeats, intervals, sprints, strides or fartlek. You can run these workouts on the track, down the road or in the woods. You don't even need a measured distance and a stopwatch; you can measure intensity by a pulse monitor or even perceived exertion. In *Run Fast,* I devoted a chapter to each of the speedwork variations, describing each in detail. In summary, though, here are the various types of speedwork and their applicability to marathon training.

Repeats. In a repeat workout, you run very fast, usually over a very short distance, and take a relatively long period of time to recover before repeating that distance. The fast (or hard) run in repeats is referred to as a repetition, or a "rep." The runner recovers almost fully between repetitions, either jogging or completely resting. When I train my high school distance runners, I have them walk a timed five minutes between reps. That allows them to recover sufficiently so they can run each repetition at near maximum speed. There's nothing magic about five minutes, but resting that precise length of time at each workout offers them a familiar landmark.

Interval training. In interval training, you carefully control the period of time, or interval, between the fast repetitions. Usually there are more reps than in repeat workouts and the distance (or time) of the interval is shorter. Key to the workout is that the heart rate is not allowed to drop too low before the runner surges into action again. Please note that the "interval" is the period *between* reps, not the repetition itself. Interval training is a more stressful form of training than most other forms of speedwork because you are never quite allowed to relax, causing a steady buildup of fatigue. For this reason, many veteran long-distance runners shy away from it.

Sprints. A sprint is just that: an all-out sprint for a short distance. The maximum distance a runner can run at full speed is probably around 300 meters, and that only if he or she is extremely well trained. Most sprints run by distance runners in practice are probably shorter than that—50 to 100 meters, a straightaway on a running track or a fairway on a golf course. The object of sprints in training is to develop style as well as speed, economy more than endurance. It's also a good way to stretch muscles and learn to lengthen your stride.

Why should a marathon runner run sprints, when at no time during the race will he or she run anywhere near that speed? The reason is that sprints develop speed. And speed is basic to success in running, regardless of your distance. If you can develop your base speed at distances of 100 meters to a mile, inevitably it will make you a faster marathon runner.

Strides. Strides are simply slow sprints. Period.

Surges. Surges are fast sprints thrown into the middle of a long run or a long race. Well, not too long a race. You probably don't surge too frequently in a marathon, or you'll surge yourself into the pickup bus for runners who can't finish. While surging at the right time might win you an Olympic medal, it's probably not a good race strategy for midpack runners whose goal is to spread their energy evenly throughout the race to maximize their performance. Nevertheless, surging is an effective and enjoyable training strategy.

Surging is also one way to get yourself out of those "bad patches" that develop in the middle of even the best-trained runner's marathon. Sometimes a surge to a slightly faster pace allows you to recover as much as if you jogged along slowly. Surges can be for any distance. Tim Nicholls, a coach from Pembroke Pines, Florida, recommends one-mile surges, as well as two-mile repeats, but a surge can be as short as 100 meters.

Fartlek. Fartlek is all of the above thrown into a single workout, usually done away from the track, preferably in the woods. It's a Swedish word that roughly translates to "speed play." Fartlek includes fast and slow running—maybe even walking. Basically, you jog or sprint or stride as the mood strikes you, generally alternating fast and slow running.

Although fartlek is best practiced on wooded trails, marathoners can adapt this type of workout to their own needs on the roads. It's an unstructured form of speed training that appeals particularly to experienced runners who have become very adept at reading their body's signals and thus don't need the discipline of a stopwatch and a measured distance.

All forms of speedwork can make you a better runner, and a better marathoner.

CHAPTER 8

Defensive Running
TECHNIQUES

W hen it comes to automobile accidents, one of the most danger-
ous spots in my hometown is on an acre of land several blocks
south of the central business district. The high-risk time is from
2:00 to about 2:15 each weekday afternoon from September
through June.

Wise people avoid the high school parking lot at this time.
Students jump in their cars and peel rubber in an attempt to
escape school as rapidly as possible.

I coach cross-country at the local high school, but I don't teach
there. I try to time my arrival either before or after the afternoon
window of madness. To do otherwise is to court disaster.

I believe in defensive driving, which is why I avoid this parking lot. I also avoid driving past taverns on Saturday nights for
fear of encountering drunk drivers. I always use my seat belt,
and my next car will have an air bag. I've looked at the statistics
about traffic accidents and know what I need to do to avoid
injury.

As a runner, I also know what I need to do to avoid injury—
not necessarily encounters with automobiles but injuries that
may be caused by overuse, training errors and so forth.

You can call these defensive running techniques. If you want
to have a long running career, you determine what activities
most often cause you to become injured, then avoid them—just
as I avoid the high school parking lot at certain times.

Are Injuries Inevitable?

Some physicians order injured runners to give up running. Several doctors offered me that advice, until I stopped going to doctors who weren't themselves runners. For most of us, stopping running permanently is not an option. We want to learn to run injury-free.

We also want to run long distances. And to run marathons is to court injury—if not from the race itself, then from the high training mileage that's necessary. Jack H. Scaff, Jr., M.D., founder of the Honolulu Marathon and director of the highly successful Honolulu Marathon Clinic, says marathon running, by definition, *is* an injury. Dr. Scaff isn't advising people not to run marathons; he's just stating what he considers a fact.

Michael L. Pollock, Ph.D., director of the University of Florida Center for Exercise Science in Gainesville, says intensity is the most common cause of running injuries. "People who only walk or jog short distances at slow paces don't become injured," says Dr. Pollock.

Stan James, M.D., the orthopedist from Eugene, Oregon, who performed orthoscopic surgery on Joan Benoit Samuelson months before her Olympic Marathon victory, claims that most running injuries are the result of "training errors." Avoid those errors, suggests Dr. James, and you can run injury-free. Lyle J. Micheli, M.D., of Boston's Children's Hospital agrees: "Many of the injuries we see could have been prevented. There is usually some type of training error."

Nevertheless, most successful training programs—including the ones presented in this book—are based on variations of the progressive overload theory. You gradually overload the system with progressively more mileage or the same mileage at faster paces. To achieve peak performance, you train to just under the point that your body would break down if you went further.

Finding Your Breaking Point

For most elite runners, this breaking point is somewhere beyond 100 weekly miles, but not everyone is blessed with superior athletic ability. Podiatrists tell us their waiting rooms are filled with average runners who run 30 miles or more a week.

Above that magic 30 miles seems to be where chondromalacia, plantar fasciitis, achilles tendinitis and other major injuries occur.

Logically, you just wouldn't run beyond that 30 miles a week, but that won't suffice for marathoners. The ideal, then, is to determine—within a tenth of a mile, if possible—the weekly mileage at which your body self-destructs. Then you can train to the edge of disaster, occasionally pushing slightly (and I emphasize the word *slightly*) over that edge to determine whether months and years of steady training (or a new pair of

Making the Most of Your Miles

Sometimes even a conservative runner who tries to ease gradually into a routine of high mileage just can't do so without injury. This is where the Unfairness Doctrine enters in.

The Unfairness Doctrine says that just when you increase quantity to the point where you feel you really are getting in shape, something happens. This is the *bête noire* of marathon running. You catch a cold. You twist an ankle. Your knee starts aching. You suffer a stress fracture.

You may be one of those people who just can't handle high mileage. If so, there are still ways to improve.

Mixing miles. In the marathoning world, this means doing different distances on different days. A runner who can't safely do more than 35 weekly miles need not run 5 miles every day, seven days a week. That runner may be able to train more efficiently by running more than 5 miles on some days and less than 5 miles on others, or even taking days off.

By altering your daily running schedule, you can increase the intensity and duration of certain workouts without necessarily increasing your weekly time commitment. (In fact, you might *save* time.)

Here is a week's training schedule that involves mixing miles.

orthotics) have allowed you to nudge your breaking point to a new level.

Pushing to that edge has to be done gradually. Elite runners spend many years gradually adapting those bodies to accept the stress of 100-mile weeks. They don't increase from 70 miles a week one month to 140 the next. A first-time marathoner who tries to double his or her weekly mileage from 35 to 70 too rapidly is likely to get into trouble.

During my second year of coaching track at our local high school, a student named Tony Morales rejoined the team midway

Sunday—15 miles
Monday—1 mile
Tuesday—10 miles
Wednesday—3 miles
Thursday—read a spy novel
Friday—6 miles
Saturday—rent a video movie: *Marathon Man*

Mixing miles is simple. But there are other ways to prevent injury and still excel in your marathon goals.

Speeding. Speeding is another variation that helps a runner improve. When you're unable to push past a certain mileage because of lack of talent, time or determination, simply run those miles faster. A runner limited to 35 weekly miles might have a training program like this.

Sunday—15 miles steady pace
Monday—2 miles recuperative jogging
Tuesday—fartlek in woods: 6 miles total
Wednesday—2 miles easy jogging
Thursday—100-yard sprints on golf course
Friday—rent a video movie: *Chariots of Fire*
Saturday—6 miles hard, or race

For real improvement, combine the principles of mixing and speeding while going farther as well.

through his junior year. He had run well as a freshman but had suffered a series of discouraging injuries and had missed most of his sophomore year.

The previous coach told me, "Tony has a lot of talent, but whenever we got his weekly mileage up over 35, he'd get injured."

"Then we'll train him at 34 miles a week," I said.

So that's what I did, and Tony was able to run pain-free. By gently pushing his limit over a period of nearly a year, Tony eventually nudged his training mileage to nearly 55 a week. As a senior, he made the All-Conference team in cross-country.

But midway through the season, Tony developed mild tendinitis in his upper thigh that limited his performance over a period of several weeks. Maybe if we had stopped at 54 miles a week, this injury would not have occurred. Or maybe not. That's the secret to injury prevention: to straddle the line between undertraining and overtraining.

Are You Overtrained?

Overtraining isn't an injury, per se. You're not hurt. Nothing is swollen, nothing is broken. You don't limp. It's just that when you train, your legs feel dead most of the time, your workout and race times have both started to deteriorate and you begin to enjoy running less and less. And you may be predisposing yourself to injury.

Marathon runners probably are more prone to overtraining than other runners, simply because of the volume of training required. It stands to reason that if you train more, you increase the chances of becoming overtrained.

Probably the key cause of the symptoms of overtraining is the loss of glycogen, the sugarlike substance that fuels your muscles and provides the readily available energy that permits them to contract efficiently. Glycogen debt can occur if you're not eating enough carbohydrates to match the amount of calories burned— or if you're not *synthesizing* enough glycogen. Excessive training appears to inhibit the body's conversion of fuel into energy, although why this occurs is not fully understood. It might be compared to having fouled sparkplugs in your automobile. The engine still runs, but not as well as it would if you bought new plugs.

The overtrained runner may maintain speed but with poorer form and with greater expenditure of energy. David Costill, Ph.D., of the Human Performance Laboratory at Ball State University in Muncie, Indiana, cited one runner who, early in his training, could run a 6:00 mile pace at only 60 percent of his aerobic capacity. Later, overtrained, the same runner had to use 80 percent of his capacity to maintain that pace.

As athletes enlist all available muscle fibers in an attempt to maintain their training pace, they invariably exhaust their fast-twitch muscles faster than their slow-twitch muscles. This is one reason runners lose speed: Their fast-twitch muscles have become exhausted through intensive training.

But glycogen depletion is not the only problem. Another is microscopic damage to the muscle fibers, which tear, fray and lose their resilience, like a rubber band that has been snapped too often. Despite analysis of blood and urine samples, researchers find it difficult to identify how, or why, chronically overtrained muscles lose their ability to contract.

Harm Kuipers, M.D., Ph.D., of the University of Limburg in the Netherlands researched the effect of overtraining for nearly a year by training racehorses on a treadmill, alternating hard days of interval sprints with easy days. Horse trainers warned that the animals would become overtrained, but this failed to happen. Finally, with time running out, Dr. Kuipers began training the horses hard on their easy days. "Almost immediately," said Dr. Kuipers, "the horses began to exhibit symptoms of being overtrained." The message to runners is: If you want to avoid overtraining, don't eliminate easy days.

Recognizing the Signs

The simplest defensive running technique you can use is your training diary. Determining where you made a mistake—that "training error" described by Dr. James—is the main reason for keeping a training diary. Learn the cause of that mistake and you are less likely to repeat it.

Your training diary can also provide clues that you're overtraining. If you've noted that you feel tired all the time, for example, you may be training too hard. "Perceived exertion may give us our most important clues," suggests William P. Morgan, Ed.D., of the University of Wisconsin in Madison.

Other symptoms to watch for:

Heavy legs. Your legs lose their snap—and speed. A run at an 8:00 pace feels like a 7:00 pace. Depleted muscle glycogen may be the cause. "You feel like you're running with glue on your shoes," says Dr. Costill.

Increased pulse rate. This is easily measured: Record your pulse each morning before you get out of bed, and cut back your training on days it's higher than usual. After doing a research project for Athletics West, Jack Daniels, Ph.D., and psychologist Scott Pengelli advised that club's athletes to cut training on days when pulse rates were high.

Sleep problems. You have trouble getting to sleep and may wake several times during the night. Then you have to drag yourself out of bed in the morning. On rising, your pulse is also elevated, as above. "Sleep dysfunctions often are a sign of overstress," says Dr. Costill.

Diminished sex drive. The romance has gone out of your life. Somehow, you seem to have lost interest in sex. Whether this is related to lowered testosterone levels caused by training, or just plain exhaustion, no one knows for sure. But overtrained runners of both sexes look and feel like zombies, says Dr. Costill.

Fear of training. You have trouble pushing yourself out the door to run each morning. So you sit and stretch longer. Your body is telling you to back off. "This is part of the psychological effect of overtraining," says Dr. Costill.

Sore muscles. Your muscles, particularly your legs, seem sore and stiff. "They may even be sore to the touch," says Dr. Costill. The reason is muscle damage, caused by too much pounding on the roads. Some muscle soreness is natural after hard training sessions, but if it persists, you're working too hard.

Former Olympic marathoner Jeff Galloway of Atlanta believes the major reason his program for training first-time marathoners succeeds is his ability to gauge the exact amount of conditioning needed to finish the event. "We have a low injury rate and folks have fun along the way," says Galloway.

Beware the Common Cold

Another early warning sign of overtraining is the common cold, particularly right before an important race.

Precompetition colds are common, claims Gregory W. Heath, D.H.Sci., an exercise physiologist and epidemiologist at the Centers for Disease Control in Atlanta. He notes that runners normally have only half as many upper respiratory infections as the general population. Up to a certain point, exercise boosts your immunity. But you lose this protection, claims Dr. Heath, if you race, and particularly if you race in marathons. David C. Nieman, D.P.H., a health professor at Appalachian State University in Boone, North Carolina, surveyed participants in the Los Angeles Marathon and found that 40 percent caught a cold during the two months before the race. By doing high-mileage training, runners lowered their resistance and became more susceptible to whatever cold bugs were floating around, even in Los Angeles's warm climate.

Dr. Nieman discovered that if runners train more than 60 miles a week, they double their risk of infection. He also found that in the week following the race, 13 percent of marathon finishers caught colds, compared with 2 percent of runners who didn't race.

It makes added sense, then, to save your high-mileage training for months when risk of infection is less (spring through fall). Also, build a strong training base so that a week lost to a cold or flu won't be a serious setback. You should start your taper early enough to prevent last-week problems. Finally, you need to be particularly wary following the race. "Spread of many viruses is hand-to-hand rather than airborne," says Heath, who recommends avoiding people with colds, washing hands after contact and particularly isolating yourself as much as possible before and after competition (avoiding crowded movie theaters, for example).

Also, cut your training during a cold and cease it entirely if you have the flu (with elevated temperature), because you may increase your chance of an injury while in a weakened condition.

Ease Into the Season

One of the first lines of defense against injuries is to quash your instinct to start training at full steam. Coaches have noted that most athletic injuries occur in the spring. "Usually I find that after a very sedentary winter, runners want to get out and start training at the same mileage level as in the fall," says one coach. "As a result, they get hurt."

Cross-training can lull you into a false sense of security. Don't overvalue off-season training that doesn't involve running. During the winter, I cross-country ski—and it gets me into fabulous cardiovascular shape. But when the snow melts, I have to be cautious about bringing the same intensity to the running trails as I did the ski trails. The one or two times I pushed right into running, I suffered injuries. In 1984, I entered several cross-country ski races in Norway, then headed south to Italy, where I ran surprisingly well in the famed Cinque Mulini race north of Milan. "Wow," I thought, "I'm in great shape." But two weeks later, I was limping.

My cardiovascular system had been in better shape than my running muscles. It was like putting a Porsche engine into a Volkswagen chassis: The chassis couldn't handle the power.

Since then I've used two strategies to help prevent this problem. First, instead of shifting completely from running to skiing as soon as snow covers the ground, I maintain a maintenance level of running, at least every other day. And once the snow melts, I cut the intensity of my training during that transition period between winter and spring.

Add Some Variety

Hector Leyba of Raton, New Mexico, a track coach and sub-3:00 marathoner, skis winters and bicycles summers. "Cross-training helps my endurance," he says. "After many years pounding the streets, I feel I need variety."

One of the main causes of running injuries is the stress caused by the literally thousands of times we hit the ground when we run. If you've ever seen any slow-motion photography of what happens to the leg muscles during a single running stride, you'd wonder how we survive even a single lap on a track, much less a marathon. Swimming, skiing, cycling and walking don't generate this ground impact, however.

It follows that if you want to maintain a high level of intensity in your training, you can shift to swimming, skiing, cycling, walking or other activities on your off days. Or select nonimpact exercises that mimic running movements. Melvin H. Williams, Ph.D., director of the Human Performance Laboratory at Old Dominion University and a top-ranked 50-plus runner, spends one day a week cross-training and does supplemental training on his off days. His one-hour off-day routine includes running in deep water wearing a flotation belt and riding standard and recumbent exercise bicycles. On the standard bike, he likes to stand up on the pedals frequently, figuring that this more closely exercises the muscles used in running, but without the impact. His recumbent workout exercises the quadriceps, sometimes overlooked in running. Again, he uses an interval approach: hard and easy.

When Dr. Williams runs less than his usual one hour, he uses cross-training to fill out the exercise period to a full 60 to 70 minutes.

Dr. Williams has selected exercises that simulate running as much as possible, but most cross-training fails to exercise the muscles *specific* to running. In order to succeed as a runner, you need to train as a runner. However, if you're prone to overuse injuries, substituting less stressful cross-training for some of your running may decrease your injuries and therefore your down time. And if you can avoid gaps in your training caused by injuries, inevitably you'll perform better as a runner.

Use Speedwork Cautiously

Every running expert I know recommends speed training as the most effective means of improving as a runner. But this can be dangerous advice if applied too zealously, particularly in training for a marathon. "Don't read what an elite athlete does in terms of mileage and attempt to do the same," advises John E. Tolbert, a coach from New Haven, Connecticut. "Get advice and train at your own level."

It isn't the speedwork itself that causes marathon runners to injure themselves in training, but speedwork coupled with the progressively longer distances run during the marathon buildup. Early in my career, I learned that I could improve either by increasing the intensity of my workouts or the distance, but I couldn't do both at the same time without risking injury. A marathoner should include speedwork in a training program only after an initial buildup to high mileage and a subsequent cutback.

In his book *Your First Marathon,* Dr. Jack Scaff, who directs the Honolulu Marathon Clinic, advised that racing or speedwork make up no more than 10 percent of your mileage. "After you've run a marathon," he warned, "you need 260 miles of training before you enter your next event, or start doing speedwork."

While I dislike formulas and don't want to suggest 10 percent as the absolute limit to speedwork—particularly because at peak training when your mileage is cut, speedwork could become a predominant part of your training—Dr. Scaff's basic advice is sound.

Choose Surfaces Carefully

I'm a believer in trail running, partly because I love to run in the woods but also because there's less chance of getting injured on the soft trail surface. Yet I notice that runners unused to varying trail surfaces face an *increased* risk of injury when they take to the woods. This happens to my cross-country team at the beginning of the fall season, or to the track team when it trains on trails after the long winter hiatus. The less dedicated runners who failed to work out off-season trip over roots or twist ankles stepping in holes, but this never seems to happen to those runners who train on trails year-round.

In addition to running trails, I like to train on the smooth fairways of golf courses. To avoid interfering with golfers, however, means getting up *very* early in the morning during the summer—a marvelous time to train if you can motivate yourself to get out of bed. Living as I do near Lake Michigan, I also find that the beach (particularly the day after high waves have flattened it) provides an ideal training surface.

In training top Dallas runners, including five-time Olympian Francie Larrieu Smith, coach Robert Vaughn avoids interval running on a track. "We do all our interval work on grass," he says. "We do repeats on the track, anything less than six reps.

Anything more, we run on grass." Since switching to grass, Vaughn has virtually eliminated the problem of stress fractures, even though his runners do two speed workouts a week.

Asphalt may be slightly less unyielding than concrete, but let's face it, neither surface is soft. Nevertheless, if you're going to race on roads, you need to train on the roads to accustom your muscles to the impact. When preparing for a marathon, I usually do a much higher percentage of my running on the roads than if I were training for shorter events, including track and cross-country races.

Footwear: Not Too Soft, Not Too Firm

One way to diminish road shock is to wear properly cushioned shoes. Running shoe companies spend millions of dollars on research and technology to design shoes that help prevent injuries. Various energy-absorbing materials and air built into or pumped into your shoes can decrease the impact of either asphalt or concrete.

One possible reason that men's marathon times have improved by nearly 20 minutes since Jim Peters's days may be better footwear and, as a result, fewer training injuries. A word of caution, however: Shoes that are *too* spongy (so soft that they offer little support) may *destabilize* the foot and become a source of injury. One shoe company in recent years came out with a marvelously comfortable shoe that was half the weight of other shoes. But the shoe was so spongy, I suspect it could contribute to injuries.

It is of paramount importance to choose your footwear *very* carefully. Among other considerations, a heavier runner will need a shoe that offers more support than a lighter runner requires. You may also need more than one type of shoe. I have a built-in rack on one basement wall where I stack my various athletic shoes, each pair for a specific purpose.

I wear heavy, protective shoes on those easy days when I run slow. When I run fast, I prefer a light shoe, and I often wear racing flats for my speed workouts and a semilight pair for long runs. When I run trails, I wear a flexible, light shoe best suited for uneven surfaces. At the track, I may don spikes for repeats. I also have cycling shoes and ski boots and Aquasocks for the beach (where I often run in deep water).

Every shoe has its own place in a runner's shoe inventory, and certain shoes that work well in one setting may not in another. Runners who wear inflexible road shoes in the woods may increase their chance of injury on the uneven ground. And while cross-training shoes may be suitable for weekend warriors who exercise infrequently, I'm not convinced they belong in the inventory of any serious endurance athlete.

When I run on grass or sand, or sometimes in deep water, I'll go barefoot, because I believe it stretches and strengthens the muscles in my feet. I've even raced without shoes à la Zola Budd Pieterse, running 5000 meters barefoot on London's Crystal Palace track in 1972 in 14:59.6, a still-standing 40-to-44 masters record for 5000 meters. That doesn't make me popular with the shoe companies, but it's all part of my defensive running approach.

Keep Muscles Loose and Strong

Stretching and strengthening is another way to minimize injury. The best time to stretch a muscle is after it's warmed up. Track runners typically jog a mile or two, then stretch or do calisthenic exercises before beginning the intense part of their workouts. That's been common practice long before Bob Anderson wrote his trend-setting best-seller, *Stretching*.

Long distance runners are less likely to pause in the middle of a long run to stretch, although this is becoming more common. Marathon coach Bill Wenmark advises several brief stretches at each water stop during a marathon. I'll stretch before long runs and in the middle of intense workouts, but my preferred time is *after* the workout, usually while relaxing in a whirlpool. Every runner should adopt a stretching regimen that is convenient and comfortable.

Strength training also is important for both conditioning and injury prevention. I lift weights and/or use exercise machines regularly in the off-season when I'm not racing regularly, but I limit strength training in the competitive season. If a specific injury threatens, I'm quick to seek advice from a trainer or physical therapist about what strength training would help.

Part of my long-term success as a runner has been avoiding those injuries that require extensive rehabilitation. During a 45-year running career, I've had very little down time. A sore Achilles tendon now and then, a strained knee once, plantar fasciitis on another occasion. Nothing much. No surgery. Either I'm smart, or lucky, or have what Dr. Costill describes as a "bulletproof body," one that is biomechanically sound. (Or it's a combination of all three.) While two of these factors are out of your control, you *can* be smart about your training by including stretching and strengthening.

To Prevent Reinjury

After suffering an injury serious enough that standard remedies such as ice and aspirin fail to provide relief, a runner needs not only to seek medical advice but also to consult his or her training diary to identify the training patterns that caused the injury.

Coming off an injury or a period of reduced training mileage, runners often reinjure themselves, claims Russell H. Pate, Ph.D., chairman of the Department of Exercise Science at the University of South Carolina. "Runners think, 'I can do 80 miles a week again,' " he says, "but their bodies aren't ready."

After following the daily training of 600 runners for a one-year period, Dr. Pate identified two major predictors for injuries: a previous injury and heavy training. "If you got injured once and don't modify your training, you probably will get injured again," says Dr. Pate.

For those doing heavy training, three factors were involved: frequency, mileage and whether or not they ran marathons. A critical problem was *approach* to training. "Too rapid a buildup is a critical factor in injuries," says Dr. Pate. "You need to know your limitations." Once you determine that, you can modify your training to prevent future injuries.

Adjust Your Program to Consider Your Age

Basic training principles apply to all runners, but specifics may vary greatly. Although running offers a marvelous means of diminishing the effects of aging, the body eventually begins to slow, and as you get older, certain cautions are in order.

Instead of one day's rest following a hard speed session or long run, you may need two days, or more. And standard training programs may not work for you if they predispose you to injury. Tom Cross, a coach from Tulsa, Oklahoma, describes a discussion he had about training with three other runners, all over 60, who had just finished an 8-K race with times faster than 35:00.

"We decided that we should just keep a steady pace and forget about the frills," says Cross. "At our age, the consensus was: Don't run intervals, don't try hills, just be consistent. Run the same every day, although the pace might vary depending on the distance. This is what older runners learn, because the secret of endurance is to stay uninjured. All you need to do is run steadily every day, and whether or not you improve, you'll at least maintain your ability as well as you can."

Rest—It's Good for You

"Dynamic repair" is a fancy title for rest coined by Bob Glover, a supervisor of coaches for the New York Road Runners Club. He considers rest to be a commonly overlooked component of any successful training program and believes that less training is sometimes best. "When in doubt, the coach should suggest less, and I've gotten softer and softer every year," he says. "By minimizing injury and getting a person to improve gradually, instead of rapidly, you'll have the most success. The old coach's mentality was to get out there and crack the whip: survival of the fittest. But how many people ended up on the junk heap along the way?"

Inevitably, if you can avoid injury, you can run long distances for the longest time. Defensive running may be the best training technique anyone can use.

CHAPTER 9

Planning for
PEAK
PERFORMANCE

Aiming at key races is the best way to achieve peak performance in long-distance events, says Russell H. Pate, Ph.D., chairman of the Department of Exercise Science at the University of South Carolina.

Yet Dr. Pate concedes that the buildup to a goal carries with it a degree of risk, which escalates as the race gets closer and the workouts more intense. "Experience indicates that high-intensity workouts are more demanding and stressful," he says. "Training hard for prolonged periods is risky in terms of overtraining and even riskier in terms of injury."

This is where progressive training aimed at a certain event—sometimes called periodization—comes in: You start from a low point of conditioning and build to a high point. You compete in a race or a series of races. You then relax your training and begin to contemplate your next goal.

More than any other event, the marathon lends itself to this approach. Although some runners—such as Doug Kurtis—run as many as a dozen marathons a year, most distance runners are content to run one or two during any given 12-month period. Usually, these races are selected well in advance, allowing ample time for a buildup to peak performance.

How do you plan for peak performance? How do you adjust your training schedule in anticipation of a specific race? How do you guarantee that you can follow that planned schedule and maximize your chances for success—and enjoyment?

"There is no magic formula," warns Keith Woodard, a coach from Portland, Oregon. "There is no magic mileage, no magic mold to put runners into. Runners are too individual for that." Nevertheless, there are certain guidelines all runners can follow to help achieve peak performance.

Timing Is Everything

If you're planning to run a marathon in the next month or so, skip ahead to the chapters on nutrition and tapering that will do you more immediate good. You don't have *time* to execute the advice that follows here. Stick a bookmark here, so you'll remember to return. After you've finished that race and have begun to plan your *next* major running campaign, read this chapter.

If you expect to peak for a specific race—whether a mile or a marathon—you need time. You need time to plan, time to establish a base, time to progress and time to taper properly.

How much time? For a short-distance event on the track or an important 5-K or 10-K on the roads, you probably need at least 3 months of preparation (although 6 months or more would be better). If you're talking marathon—not one you enter casually, but one you really focus on—6 months is probably minimum, and 12 would be better. Those with Olympic aspirations must think four years ahead. I planned 18 months ahead for one of my best races, a sub-2:30 marathon I ran to win a gold medal at the 1981 World Veterans Championships in New Zealand. And as an aging veteran, I'm already contemplating races I might run in the next century.

Doug Renner, a coach from Westminster, Maryland, suggests you develop a two- to four-year game plan. "Goals must continually be refined," Renner says. "Runners need to know the big picture, rather than just haphazardly go from race to race."

You want enough time to execute a well-organized plan that will bring you to the starting line in the best shape of your life. If you don't do that, you're not peaking.

Why You Need a Goal

Before you make a plan, you need a goal. "The ability to adhere to a specific well-thought-out and long-term training program is the most necessary factor leading to success in the marathon," advises Clark Campbell, a coach and professional triathlete from Lawrence, Kansas.

In other words, when you have no destination, any road will take you there. If you want to float along from week to week, training the way you feel, racing whenever you want to, that's fine. Running need not always be a relentless pursuit of one Big Event after another. We all need down time to renew ourselves psychologically, to gather ourselves for the next push. Sometimes I'll take a year or more off from serious training and racing. I've spoken often about the Bowerman approach that features hard days and easy days; I'll often plan hard years and easy years. But *not* having a goal might even be considered having a goal.

Usually I set goals at the beginning of each year, when I'm starting a new diary. Sometimes my goals will be a set of times I want to better at various distances—or maybe there are a number of races I want to do well in. Most frequently, I attempt to peak for the World Veterans Championships, which comes at two-year intervals. Other times, I'll peak for a marathon.

Marathons lend themselves to goal-setting, because of the extra effort required to both train for them and to compete well in them—plus the magic of the marathon itself. One of my sidelines over the last dozen years has been leading groups for Roadrunner Tours to distance running events. I learned early on that it was difficult to coax people to shorter distance events, such as the 12-K Bay-to-Breakers Run in San Francisco or the 15-K City-to-Surf Run in Sydney, Australia. We got so few takers, we had to cancel our plans. But Athens or Honolulu for a marathon? "Sign me up!" It seems that when people lay out more than $1,000 for a running vacation, they want to go the full 26.2 miles.

But setting a goal involves not merely selecting an event or events but also deciding what you expect from your participation in that event. Is your goal just to finish? Is your goal a PR? Is your goal victory—or at least placing high in your age group? Or maybe you're just out to have a good time? Once your principal goal is determined—and only after that—can you begin to make plans.

It is also possible to have subgoals, or a series of goals. You may want to run some preliminary races—and run them well— as interim contests before the main race that interests you most. Sometimes I select a primary goal (such as running a fast marathon), expecting to use it as a stepping stone to a greater goal (running a faster marathon). Doug Kurtis says, "Marathoners need short-term goals, other races leading up to the marathon. I'm amazed when I meet people and their first race is a marathon. It's hard to focus on a marathon two or three months away, so focusing two or three weeks ahead on a 10-K can help keep you motivated."

On the other hand, if your goals are too many or too diverse, you may have difficulty achieving your main goal, which defeats the purpose.

Developing Your Game Plan

Once you set your goal, you can make a *plan* to achieve that goal. Here's where old training diaries come in handy, particularly for those of us who have been running more than a few years. Whether or not I actually pull individual diaries down from the shelf or not, I'll at least mentally review what has worked in the past and what hasn't. Even if I decide to take a totally different approach—say, low-mileage training instead of high-mileage—it will be pursued after considerable reflection.

I do a lot of my preliminary planning on airplanes returning from major events. If, as so often happens, it's an overseas flight, I have plenty of time trapped in a tight seat with nothing better to do than think. Invariably the food is terrible and I've already seen what is probably a bad movie, so what better time for considering what next to achieve? Sometimes I'll pull out a notebook and jot down dates and times. Or I'll tap away at my laptop computer, which I frequently take with me on trips.

Inevitably, however, I fine-tune my plan after returning home. On a large sheet of poster board, I draw a home-made calendar with large blocks for each date. I'll list major events in appropriate boxes, usually drawing a red border around *the* important box, the day on which I want to hit my peak. I may list certain workouts I want to run, or distances (daily or weekly) I want to achieve. Or I use the calendar to record how my training is going. I'll record the distance of my long runs and my weekly miles. Key speed workouts may be plotted in advance or recorded after they occur. The same with races and times at those races. (This is in addition to my regular diary, where every day I record more specific detail about individual workouts.)

Planning is where time and goal come together. If you have a specific period of time in which to achieve a specific goal, you can plan accordingly—to a point, of course. You can't predict whether the wind will be in your face or the weather will be too warm. But you can plan almost every other aspect of your marathon training so you'll reach the starting line ready to perform to the best of your ability.

If you can plan to achieve that, it won't matter how fast you run or whom you beat.

In an article I wrote for *Runner's World,* Dr. Pate advised, "Figure out the key sessions you need for your program. Get them in there, then surround them with those kind of recovery activities that allow you to continue over a period of time. Build your program on priorities. The highest priority is attached to the key, hard sessions.

"The secret to success in long-distance running is not what type of workouts you do, whether high or low intensity, but how those workouts are structured into a specific program and incorporated throughout a training year—and for the length of a career as well."

You might want to reread that paragraph. It may be the most important message you encounter in this book.

Taking Time Off

How important is rest? It's more important than most of us realize, says Paul Goss, a top-ranked duathlete and coach from Foster City, California.

While you're choosing your goal and planning your attack, you may want to take time to relax: a planned vacation, not necessarily away from running, but away from training at maximum effort. *Rest* is a word you have encountered before in this book, and it is a word you will encounter again.

Rest isn't always entirely optional, of course. If you've completed a marathon, you may be forced into a period of recuperation that could last a week, a month, or more. This time is necessary not only to allow sore muscles to recover but also to permit rejuvenation of the spirit.

The spirit may take more time for recovery than the muscles. Psychiatrists talk about postmarathon depression. Usually there is a period of well-deserved euphoria following a peak performance, particularly one involving much preparation. First-time marathoners are more susceptible than others because they have passed—for better or worse—through a unique experience. They wonder: "What do I do next?" and often there is no immediate answer.

One year, Ron Gunn of Southwestern Michigan College and I took a large number of runners from his beginning running class to the Honolulu Marathon. The morning after the race, we planned a short walk from our hotel to the Royal Hawaiian Hotel on the beach for brunch. Nearly everybody appeared wearing the "finisher" shirt they had won the previous day. Inevitably, of course, that revered shirt gets thrown into the dirty laundry.

Regardless of whether or not you immediately select your next goal, take ample time to rest before setting out to achieve it.

Stabilize Your Training

In many respects, the base period is an extension of the rest period. Usually within a week after finishing a marathon, muscle soreness will almost completely disappear and you can begin to run comfortably again. But you need time to stabilize your training. Don't rush immediately into all-out training aimed at your next goal. If you do, you're liable to crash some weeks or months later.

Everybody has a comfortable base level of training, a weekly maintenance mileage that he or she can accomplish almost effortlessly. For me, this base level is about 25 or 30 miles. I don't have to aim at running that far; it just happens. If I'm just going out the door five or six days a week without thinking about where I'm going or how far or how fast, I'll end the week with this level. That's my base maintenance level to which I return periodically: It's enough to maintain a reasonable percentage of my peak fitness level.

While training at this level, I often cross-train. If I've just finished a fall marathon, I'll swing eagerly into the cross-country ski season. I'll also spend more time lifting weights, since inevitably I will have eliminated strength training during my final race countdown.

I rarely peak for winter events, but after a spring marathon, I might do some cycling or swimming, compete in some triathlons or run some summer 10-K races—which I like because hot weather offers you a built-in excuse for slow times. I'll sometimes run these races on impulse, only deciding to enter on race morning.

Quite often, my peak performances are keyed to late-summer track meets. Once past the track season, I divert time and energy in the fall to road races such as the Scenic Ten (ten miles) in Park Forest, Illinois, or the Blueberry Stomp (15-K) in Plymouth, Indiana. Last fall, I ran a 25-K along a towpath beside the I&M Canal near Channahon, Illinois, and that's a race I would love to include on my annual schedule. I may run a fall marathon with minimal preparation, with no goal other than that of having a good time.

Running many different races can take the edge off this period of base training, but the important point is to slack off and give yourself some time when you're not too serious about anything connected with running—either racing or training. When it comes time to concentrate your training toward a peak goal, you move into a new phase.

Racking Up the Miles

Practically every beginner's program depends on gradually increasing distance, usually weekly and on the day you do your longest run. Nobody's been able to come up with a better program, and I doubt anybody ever will. It's the old story of Milo (the ancient Greek wrestler) and the bull. You start lifting a calf when it is young, and by the time the calf grows into a heavy bull, you have the strength to throw people out of the ring in the Olympics.

The same with running: You take people running 25 miles a week, and by adding a few miles a week over a period of three months, you get them up near 50 miles weekly. You take people capable of running an hour (or about 8 miles) continuously and help them to progress to where they can run for three hours (or about 20 miles).

If you're talking *peak* performance, however, you need to do more than spend 12 weeks adding a mile a week and increasing your final long workout to 20 miles. You need to take sufficient time (or have a sufficient base) to arrive at that level probably at least two *months* before the marathon—and hold at that level.

A single 20-miler isn't enough. For peak performance, you need to develop the ability to run 20-milers repeatedly (two or three times a month) without undue fatigue and without becoming overtrained.

Some runners go beyond marathon distance in their training. At one period I progressed to 31-mile workouts, but eventually I decided that it was counterproductive, at least for me. It took too much time, and I had to slow down too much to achieve that distance. During peak marathon training, however, I add a second semilong run to my training week, usually about two-thirds of the distance of the long run: 10 miles if my long run is 15; 13 to 15 miles if my long run is 20. It's possible to increase your long and semilong runs simultaneously, but a more sensible approach is to stabilize your long run near 20, then begin a progression featuring a second workout.

Don't forget that word I promised to use again in this chapter: *rest.* Every third or fourth week, depending on how I feel, I take an extra day or two of rest. I back down from my weekly mileage and maybe skip my long run that week. That allows me to gather strength so that I can progress to a still higher level.

Pumping Up the Intensity

Another standard approach for elite runners is to increase the intensity of their training sessions. One way to increase overall intensity is to do your long runs faster. When I peak for spring marathons, this happens naturally. As the weather warms, I can run more fluidly in shorts and a T-shirt than I can in the multi-layered outfit I wear in colder weather. Similarly, before fall marathons, I find I can run more comfortably (and faster) as the weather cools, at least to a point. Some natural speeding is acceptable as you increase distance and improve fitness, but to push too fast, too far, too soon raises the specter of overtraining and injury.

A better approach is to run distance workouts at a steady pace and to increase intensity in separate speed sessions. In fact, most experienced runners decrease their mileage at least slightly when moving from the distance phase to speed phases of their peak training plans. Various forms of speedwork, particularly interval training, lend themselves to progressive training of this sort.

A typical speed progression would be to start with running 10 × 400 in 75 seconds with a 400 jog between, then over ten successive weeks lower the time one second a week until you are capable of running 10 × 400 in 65 seconds. Such a progression works only if you begin conservatively, however, and don't pick an end goal beyond your capabilities. Another approach would be to begin at 5 × 400 and add an extra repetition at the same pace each week until you achieve 10 × 400, or more.

But don't make the mistake I once made when I increased speed and number simultaneously. While training in Germany in 1956, I began at 10 × 400 in 70 seconds and tried to add a 400 a week and drop a second a week. A few weeks before reaching my goal of 20 × 400 in 60 seconds, I suffered a sudden drop in performance.

Hills Fulfill a Purpose

Hill training is another means of increasing intensity. You can run sprints up hills as a form of speed training or shift to hilly courses for your long runs. Preparing for the Sunburst Marathon, which has a relatively flat course, I also selected flat courses for my long runs. If I were preparing for a hillier marathon, such as Boston, I would probably train over hillier courses, at least during the closing stages of my training.

Because Joe Catalano coaches in New England, where the Boston Marathon is the annual focus of many runners, he has his athletes do their long workouts on hilly courses, feeling that the combination of hills and distance increases endurance. "Many people shy away from hills," says Catalano, "especially when they go long. They make it easy on themselves—but that limits their improvement. It's a matter of strength: The more you repeat something, the stronger you get. We run long every week for best results. Wait more and you fail to improve. We start novice runners on courses as short as 3 to 6 miles. Very gradually we build: 8, 10, 12, 14, 16, then level off. We'll start on a series of small hills spaced apart. Then as the runners get stronger, we seek steeper hills closer together." One advantage of the Boston area, he says, is that it's fairly hilly.

The advantage of training using an overload, or progressive, period similar to that proposed by Catalano is that as you get tougher, you toughen the workout. This provides a strong psychological "carrot" for the runner trying to peak for a specific race. After the long runs to develop endurance, after the fast runs to develop strength, you use a shot of speed training to fine-tune your speed.

Consider Other Factors

Blind application of any number-based system can cause problems. One variable not mentioned in many coaching articles is weather. Whether it's cold or hot, windy or rainy, can affect how fast or how far you run during any given workout. The number of miles you have run doesn't necessarily reflect the quality of your training.

Top masters runner Barry Brown is an investment consultant who commutes by air between offices in Bolton Landing, New York, and Gainesville, Florida. Brown trains with a pulse monitor so he can measure the relative intensity of workouts, regardless of variables.

He once described to me one interval workout featuring mile repetitions, which he ran averaging 5:20 per mile in cool weather in New York, then averaged 5:40 in hot weather in Florida the following week. "The intensity measured by my pulse rate was exactly the same," he told me. "But if you just looked at the numbers in my diary, you would have thought I was taking it easy in the second workout."

Fatigue, diet and sleep all can affect the intensity of your training. Monitoring intensity is probably the trickiest aspect of any training program, even for an experienced runner, and is one reason a knowledgeable coach can help you shave minutes off your marathon time. Self-trained runners who are well motivated can too easily get themselves in trouble. If they train in a group, where group dynamics sometimes take precedence over good sense, they can suffer similar problems.

For the above reasons, I do not recommend doing interval training—or any form of speedwork—year-round. However, it's a type of training that lends itself well to progressing toward a specific goal.

Reviewing the Plan

At various points during the premarathon buildup, I like to review what I am doing. Am I on schedule? Am I training too hard and need to back off? What level of fitness have I achieved and how will that affect my pace in the marathon?

In some respects, this review is ongoing, because every day on my way out to train I pass my training calendar on the wall, where I can see at a glance the number of weekly miles I've run and the distance of my long runs, and whether I'm on schedule or not. My smaller diary provides me with the details of my training and I sometimes thumb backward through it if I'm planning to progress in certain workouts (either in distance or intensity). I also look for key words, such as "tired," or "dragging," or "legs dead," which, if they occur too often, are a clear signal to me that I need several easy days or a week of low mileage to avoid injury or overtraining.

During any review, I'll decide only to *decrease* the level of my training; I never decide to *increase* that level. If you think you're behind your premarathon schedule, you either need to lower your performance expectations or choose another race later in the year.

One way to determine your fitness level is to enter a race over a well-established distance. It's easy enough to find a 10-K race to jump into, although I would prefer to test myself at either a ten-miler or a half-marathon. A 25-K would be ideal, but there are only a few of those around. (One of the best in my area is the Old Kent River Bank Run in Grand Rapids, Michigan, although its mid-May date eliminates it as preparation for most spring marathons.)

I don't like to race too often during my peak buildup for any major event, but particularly not before a marathon. To race properly, I find I need to rest several days before the race, and it takes me several days afterward to recover. Before you know it, you've lost the equivalent of a week of productive training. For that reason I try to limit any test races in the premarathon buildup to one a month.

Your time in test races can help you predict your marathon time and guide you in pace selection. But in making comparisons, beware of overconfidence. You also may need to adjust depending on conditions, including weather and difficulty of the course. Leading up to the Sunburst Marathon, I planned a final test in Kalamazoo, Michigan, at 15-K.

Alas, race day dawned wet and cold and the course had several hills that slowed my pace accordingly. I also had run too hard doing mile repeats in practice a few days earlier. In Kalamazoo, I couldn't even equal my practice pace, which was discouraging for someone who prides himself on performing best when it counts. Still, the combination of tough workouts and a decent race under atrocious conditions told me I was at least moving forward toward my goals. (But I cut my mileage the following week to prevent overtraining.)

The Reward: The Peak

Eventually, if you have planned well, you reach a peak in your training. Running becomes easier and less of an effort. You are able to finish your weekly long runs at the same pace you started—and you don't feel as tired or worn out the next day. If you are running speedwork on the track, your times are faster. You feel good. You look lean and mean. One of the best indicators of my fitness level was when my wife's mother would look at me and say, "You're too skinny!" It was then that I knew I was in shape.

All of the above offers positive feedback and will provide a psychological boost when you run your big race. If you know you're in shape, you're more likely to feel confident that you can achieve a peak performance. A classic example from my own career occurred in 1975 as I was driving from the hotel to the track in Toronto where I would run the 3000-meter steeplechase in the 1975 World Veterans Championships. A black cat dashed in front of my car. "Good!" I thought. "I'm going to prove just how silly superstition is."

I won the race that evening by outkicking two runners from Australia and New Zealand in the last lap: a victory for positive thinking and peak planning. To achieve peak performance, mental strength may be as important as physical strength, but you achieve mental confidence by training yourself physically.

Most first-time marathoners train to reach a quick peak—that final 20-miler before the race. But if they're well coached, they won't try to achieve a peak performance in their first marathon, saving that for later races.

Most experienced marathoners like to reach a peak, then hold that training level for four to six weeks. Once you get to the point where you have the time and ability to run several 20-milers, you are more likely to achieve the peak performance you want. You will also probably chop minutes off the time you ran in that first marathon.

One approach, popularized by the New Zealand coach Arthur Lydiard, is to build a strong mileage base, then shift to speedwork for fine-tuning in the last month of training, reducing mileage slightly to compensate for the intensity of the faster training. This approach has worked for me and for many other distance runners.

But Steve Spence, bronze medalist in the marathon at the 1991 World Championships, took an opposite approach. He did his speedwork early during the base training period, then switched to long distance during the final month before the race. He was guided by David E. Martin, Ph.D., an adviser to the U.S. Olympic Committee. Gelindo Bordin, the 1988 Olympic champion, reportedly used a similar approach in his training. This method, however, may better serve a highly conditioned, elite athlete who rarely strays far from peak performance than the rest of the running world.

The Final Taper

The final touch to any program designed to achieve peak performance is the taper, the gradual cutback of training that occurs immediately before the race. This is so important a subject that I've devoted all of the next chapter to it.

The one factor critical to your taper is rest, something many dedicated runners have trouble doing. You need to arrive at the starting line Rested, Refreshed and Ready to run, the three Rs of peak performance. But more on this in the following chapter.

CHAPTER 10

The
MAGIC TAPER

After months and months of train-ing, after the steady buildup of weekly miles and a string of long runs on weekends, the big event is near. Many questions may spring to mind: What do you do the last week or two before the marathon? How do you pre-pare yourself physically and mentally? How much should you rest? How do you cut back on training, or taper? How *long* should you taper?

This is when many marathoners make a serious mistake. They fail to utilize one key ingredient in any training system that's mentioned many times in this book: *rest.*

Fear of Tapering

David L. Costill, Ph.D., of Ball State University, believes that runners often train too hard in the weeks immediately preceding a marathon. "They feel they need one last butt-busting workout and end up tearing themselves down," says Dr. Costill.

Runners rarely taper, or cut back their training, for more than a week, even for a major marathon. But in his research with swimmers, Dr. Costill noticed that they often set PRs by tapering as much as three to six weeks before an event.

He also found that swimmers performed better when under-trained. So when Dr. Costill worked with a group of runners, he started their taper three weeks before a track race. During this period they ran only two easy miles daily.

Two problems developed. Psychological tests showed that the runners, addicted to running and worried about losing conditioning, became anxious. Also, in a preliminary 5000-meter trial, the runners—apparently so well rested they misjudged their abilities—went out too fast and faded at the end. But in a subsequent trial, the runners paced themselves and ran their best times.

Dr. Costill eventually concluded that runners can best achieve success in long-distance running by preparing far in advance. "Base is important," he says. "Runners need to start their marathon training early enough so that they can afford to taper two or three weeks before the event. You need to realize that it is the training you do *months* before—rather than weeks before— that spells success."

That's a message we all should heed, but the drive that pushes us to success often pushes us to train too hard at the end. This is particularly true of seasoned marathoners. We become comfortable with our regular training routine, whether it's 40, 50, 60 or more weekly miles, and don't *want* to cut back.

We may not know what to do with the extra time. And we don't want to give up our long Sunday run with friends, even the last weekend before the marathon. Then there's the problem of diet. If you cut the number of miles, you'll also need to cut the number of calories you eat if you don't want to gain weight. And while many marathoners might believe that rest could benefit their performance in *this* marathon, they're afraid of the effect of two or three weeks' rest on their overall conditioning.

Cut Back—It's *Good* for You

Nevertheless, if you want to run well in the marathon, you need to change habits in four areas.

Cut total mileage. Many of us are slaves to our training logs. We find security in the consistency with which we run week after week, month after month, recording a steady succession of miles in our diaries and on our calendars. That's fine, since steady and consistent training brings results, but for the last two to three weeks before the marathon, mileage doesn't count. In fact, high mileage may hinder your performance.

According to Owen Anderson, Ph.D., editor of *Running*

Research News, "Scientific evidence suggests that temporary training reductions bolster leg muscle power, reduce lactic acid production and carve precious minutes off race times. In contrast, hard workouts just before a race can produce nagging injuries and deplete leg muscles of their key fuel for running—glycogen."

How much should you cut mileage? That's a tough question, because we all are different and our goals differ. As a general rule, I'd say cut total mileage by at least 50 percent, and later in this chapter I'll present specific programs for how to do this.

Cut frequency. The simplest way to cut total mileage is to reduce the number of times you train. When I was training at the elite level and running twice a day, I cut my mileage by eliminating one of those daily workouts the last ten days before a race.

You may not train twice daily, but if you follow a hard/easy pattern in your training, you have a similar option. Just eliminate the easy days. Instead of running an easy five-miler on your in-between days, don't run at all. Take a day off. You'll allow your body to recover more fully from the hard workouts, and you won't lose any conditioning.

Cut distance, not intensity. Research suggests that you need to continue to train at or near race pace on those hard days. At McMaster University in Hamilton, Ontario, a group led by Duncan MacDougall, Ph.D., compared different ways of tapering in well-trained runners who averaged 45 to 50 miles a week. For the taper week, some athletes didn't run, others ran 18 to 19 miles at an easy pace, and another group cut their mileage but continued running fast. The researchers decided that a taper including small amounts of fast running was superior to slow, easy miles.

Dr. MacDougall also worked with runners training for a 10-K race who started their taper with 5 × 500 at race pace, then progressively eliminated one 500 for the next five days, ending with a one-day rest.

Dr. MacDougall commented: "We still don't know what the optimal tapering plan actually is, but we do know that if you're going to be tapering for a week or so, it's important to keep the intensity of your workouts fairly high as you cut back drastically on your mileage."

Translated to the marathon, this would mean maintaining the pace of your runs but cutting their distance. A hard eight-mile run would become a six-mile run at the beginning of the taper, then later get cut to four or two. But you should keep the pace near the comfortable pace you've used for most of your training. In speed workouts, cut the number of repetitions similar to the McMaster's taper.

Finally, watch what you eat. If you're running less, you're also burning fewer calories. This could mean you gain a pound or so—no big deal, unless you also fill in your spare time by making extra trips to the fridge.

Robert Eslick, a coach from Nashville, Tennessee, says, "I tell my runners to watch their intake for the first three days of the marathon week to avoid weight gain and then to eat a little more than their normal intake, with the emphasis on carbohydrates, the last three days."

To keep from piling on extra pounds, you could eliminate junk foods from your regular diet during your tapering week. Get rid of the soft drinks and sugar sweets that you may have used to *boost* your calorie intake during regular training. Rely on complex carbohydrates instead—potatoes, apples, pasta, bread and so on.

Tapering Formulas That Work

Knowing precisely how to modify your training during the last two to three weeks before a marathon takes experience. Even for seasoned marathoners it may take a few bad starts before finding a specific routine that works. There are too many variables in the equation: how long you may have prepared for any one specific long race, how effective your training has been, whether you enter the closing stages undertrained or overtrained and how confident you are.

A good coach familiar with your abilities and training patterns can tell you how to taper. If any one of the more than 50 coaches who completed questionnaires for this book worked with you on a day-by-day basis, he or she could tell you precisely how to modify your training for the final countdown. Or if these experienced coaches reviewed your training diary, they could tell you how to taper. They might tell you to run eight miles this day and four miles that, and rest the third.

A general training plan is vital six months before the race, and a specific tapering plan three weeks before can help you reap the results of your long training buildup. Here is how you should approach that final period before the marathon.

Week three: Three weeks (21 days) before the race, you need to begin at least thinking about your taper. Ideally, this is a week when you *stabilize* your training. If you planned properly, the previous week should have been your high point in mileage, intensity or both. Most experienced runners plan to peak with three weeks to go. You should avoid the trap of thinking that one additional week of training just might get you in really good shape. It's more likely to injure you or lower your resistance so you're at risk of catching a cold or the flu—a big liability when you have a race to run.

You can run as hard this week as you did the week before, but no harder. If it's the week for your final 20-miler, resist the temptation to push to 21 or 22. If your weekly mileage last week was 50, keep it there. *Don't* try for 55.

But most runners will benefit by a slight decrease in their mileage, to about 75 percent of the mileage the week before. The runner who ran 50 miles last week should cut back to somewhere between 35 and 40 miles. An easy way to cut total mileage is to convert one or two of your easy days into rest days. Change one or two others into half workouts, decreasing your distance. But don't yet cut intensity or pace. You can cut the number of your repeats during speed workouts, for example, but don't run them slower.

Week two: If you *didn't* cut mileage last week, cut it now. You need at least ten days to taper. If you feel you must run a final 20-miler two weeks before the race, it should be your final workout at this distance.

If you did cut your mileage to 75 percent last week, now you should cut it to nearly 50 percent of your normal mileage. The marathoner who normally runs 50 miles a week should now run 25 miles.

Here's where you begin to reduce intensity by cutting back on your long runs. You should decrease your 20-mile run to 12 to 16 miles, and cut the distance on your other fast runs as well. But don't yet reduce your pace. You don't want to forget too soon what it feels like to train at near-marathon pace.

Remember that along with the decreased mileage, you'll be burning fewer calories, so if you're worried about gaining a pound or two, cut back on your intake of "empty" calories.

Week one: If you've *resisted* the idea of cutting your mileage before, at least cut it now. Even macho, supermileage, another-lap-around-the-park, give-me-100 zealots will concede that maybe a little taper is helpful at this point. Okay, if you wouldn't taper for three weeks, how about three days? Did you really believe running 20 miles the final Sunday before your race was going to help you?

Speaking of diet, begin carbo-loading seven days in advance. Forget what you read years ago about depletion and three days of a low-carbohydrate diet before switching to a diet high in carbohydrates. Stick with a high-carbohydrate diet throughout the week. You don't need to eat spaghetti all seven days: Focusing on fruits, vegetables and grains will keep you above 60 percent carbos even if you have lean meat as a main course. If you haven't eliminated between-meal junk snacks, do it now.

This is also the week to *eliminate* hard training. There's no room in your training plan for hard, fast or long runs. Forget them. If you run anything at or near race pace, don't run far. I enjoy doing "strides," which are sprints at race pace. But by definition, strides are short: 150 meters at the most. Soft surfaces are best. Instead of jogging between, I'll walk.

And now is not the time to cross-train. According to Tom Grogon, a coach from Cincinnati, Ohio, "One problem that often develops is that people in training sometimes use these easy/lower mileage weeks to do something else equally stressful." Grogon recalls one tapering runner who rebuilt his barn and another who spent his "rest" time swimming and biking—and none of these activities exactly qualify as *resting*. He recommends using the extra time to catch up on family and work responsibilities.

Days three to one: For the final three days of the countdown, I shift to almost total rest. Notice I said "almost." During the final three days, I rest two, run one. This is my usual pre-marathon pattern:

Three days before is a day off.

Two days before is a day off.

One day before, I may do some light jogging and perhaps do a few strides, particularly if I've traveled a long distance to the race.

If possible, I prefer to travel at least two days before the race, not the day before. Travel fatigues me, and I prefer to get to the race city early. For international races requiring an overnight jet flight, I need to arrive *much* earlier. For a short overseas track race, I'll sometimes arrive a couple of days before I compete; for marathons, I need nearly a week to adjust. One rule of thumb is to arrive one day early for every time zone crossed—if the cost of hotel rooms doesn't prohibit it. Ask yourself: How important is this race? Then plan accordingly.

24 hours: The important point to remember about the last 24 hours is that if you have prepared properly, nothing much you do on this day—except what you eat and drink—will have much effect on your race. As for training, if what you do allows you to relax—including those strides mentioned earlier—do it. Mental preparation is probably more important than physical preparation at this point.

One way to pass time the day before the race is to hang out at the exhibition of running equipment that's as much a part of the marathon mystique as the pasta party. But don't spend all day on your feet, particularly on the hard concrete in most exhibition halls. If you want to chat with your friends, do it in your room or sitting in soft chairs in the lobby.

Another option is touring the course. A number of coaches responding to my questionnaire felt it important that their runners see the course in advance, so they know what to expect.

But having been in the running business this long as a runner and as a reporter, I've either run over most of the courses I race or ridden them on press trucks. I don't need to see them one more time, or even *one* time, particularly if it means committing myself to sitting for several hours on a bus. With several thousand people around you on race day, you're not going to get lost.

To me the hills always seem steeper and the miles longer when you're riding over them rather than running them. But if there are key points of a course I feel I need to see—such as a series of hills—I might make an effort to see them, but usually I'm content to wait until race day.

The Final Feast

My all-time favorite running book title is *Spaghetti Every Friday,* written by Houston runner Bob Fletcher, who ran 50 marathons on 50 successive weekends. (And your spouse considers *you* obsessive.) This title refers to the ritual spaghetti dinner the night before most major marathons. Often you can eat on the cheap at these affairs, but sometimes they're noisy and impersonal. My nominee for the best prerace pasta party is the Chicago Marathon, but Motor City (Detroit) comes close.

To avoid crowds, I'll sometimes sneak off to a local Italian restaurant—if I can find one without a 30-minute wait. Or I may pick a Chinese restaurant where I can eat a rice dish.

Wherever or whatever you eat, your last meal needs to be high in carbohydrates. But don't overeat, thinking more is better. The night before the 1982 Avon Women's International Marathon in San Francisco, I sat next to a top runner who piled a world-record amount of pasta on her plate. Then she went back for seconds!

She was only 5 feet 5 inches tall and weighed 109 pounds, so I don't know where she stored all that food. And I don't recall that she ran too well the next day.

Basically, don't eat any more at the prerace pasta party than you're used to. Eat a normal-sized meal and drink what you usually drink. Most experts advise against beer, because it's a diuretic, but if you're used to having an occasional beer with your meal and you think it will relax you, it probably will.

Research at Ball State University suggests that eating two small meals four hours apart the night before the race may be better than eating one larger meal. Dr. Costill suggests that a high-carbohydrate snack just before going to bed may help assure a full supply of glycogen in your muscles. You should, however, avoid soft drinks with caffeine that may keep you awake. My caffeine limit is normally one cup of coffee or one soft drink, but I won't even have that the night before a marathon.

With or without caffeine in my system, I may sleep fitfully or awaken in the middle of the night. This used to worry me; it no longer does. I thought I was losing energy by lying awake in bed, but as long as you're horizontal you're still getting rest. More important than the night before is the night *before* the night before. For a Sunday race, make certain you sleep well on Friday, and don't worry about Saturday.

One final item in my premarathon countdown: I always pin my number on my singlet before I go to bed. In deference to the sponsors, I no longer fold around the numeral to cut wind resistance, but I will fold the bar strip under. I usually bring extra safety pins in case there aren't enough in my race packet, as I don't want the number flapping in the wind.

With my singlet so pinned—and I'll try it on to make certain I haven't pinned the front to the back—I'll position it on a chair in my hotel room along with my shorts, warmup clothes and any other gear, with my shoes (socks inside) positioned under the chair pointing in the right direction as though I were seated in the chair. I once felt somewhat foolish doing this, but I've talked to enough other runners to now realize I am not alone.

When it comes to the marathon, you don't want to leave anything to chance.

CHAPTER 11

The
DISTANCE
RUNNER'S DIET

I t was tough for those of us who ran long distance in the 1960s. We were poorly served nutritionally because of our own lack of knowledge and an equal lack among event organizers. We didn't know what to drink—or *whether* to drink. Race officials rarely provided fluids on the course and frequently scheduled starting times so we ran during the hottest part of the day. Our motto could have been: "Mad dogs and marathoners go out in the midday sun."

Somehow we survived, and the sport began to prosper—but only after major changes were made in the distance runner's diet.

The Dark Ages of Sports Nutrition

A page from my 1963 training diary is particularly frightening. While being coached by Fred Wilt, I kept meticulous records of everything from temperature and humidity to what I ate. It was June 30, at the National Amateur Athletic Union (AAU) 25-Kilometer Championships in Detroit, Michigan. The race started at 1:30 in the afternoon. It was 94°; the humidity was high and there wasn't a cloud in the sky. I recorded the weather as "hot!!" There was no drinking water on the course past ten miles.

Most astounding was my prerace meal. For breakfast at 7:30 A.M., I had orange juice and cereal, which was a good start, but my choices for lunch several hours later seem strange today. I had more orange juice, bread, milk and a *6-ounce steak!* Little wonder I suffered problems that day. I kept pace for half the distance with eventual winner Peter McArdle of the New York Athletic Club, then faded badly to barely salvage third.

Fred Wilt and I knew even then that good nutrition was essential for success in endurance events, but we hadn't yet fitted together all the puzzle pieces. I usually had problems in the closing stages of marathons because I ran out of energy, so I experimented with various nutritional means of boosting energy stores. At various times, I taped dextrose tablets to the back of my shorts to take during the race, or drank a high-energy drink called Sustagen, a milkshake-like supplement often used for the elderly. It made me belch through the first half of the Boston Marathon one year without helping much the second half.

Actually, where diet was concerned, some of the veteran runners from New England knew better. In the 1950s, New England was a hotbed of roadrunning activity. In fact, it was the *only* bed. When I first arrived at Boston in 1959, I learned that the traditional breakfast for marathoners was "porridge," what I knew as oatmeal. I made fun of this strange New England meal in an article I wrote called "On the Run from Dogs and People" for *Sports Illustrated* (which I later expanded into a book with the same title) before the 1963 Boston Marathon.

I should have kept my mouth shut. Or rather opened it, and started to eat. Oatmeal is high in carbohydrates and, sweetened with honey and coupled with orange juice, was exactly the kind of premarathon meal I should have been eating.

Getting a Handle on Nutrition

By the end of the decade, we began to get an idea of what diet worked best for distance runners. David L. Costill, Ph.D., established the Human Performance Laboratory at Ball State University in Muncie, Indiana, in 1966, and I became one of his first guinea pigs. One of his early experiments involved fluid replacement. One summer, I ran two hours on a treadmill on three successive days in Dr. Costill's lab—the equivalent of three 20-milers—drinking either nothing, water or Gatorade.

When allowed to drink at the rate of 50 milliliters every five minutes, my core body temperature remained several degrees lower than when running without fluids. The replacement drink provided a glucose boost that theoretically would permit me to run cooler and faster.

Dr. Costill continued his research on race nutrition. Within a few years, in some of the earliest experiments on carbohydrate loading, his assistant Bill Fink was cooking large pots of spaghetti in the Ball State lab to feed to runners. The word soon leaked out to the sports world: Steaks were out, pasta was in. Several years later, I had an assignment to write an article for the *New York Times Magazine* on a quarterback for the Kansas City Chiefs. I noted with interest that Hank Stram, coach of the Chiefs, was already promoting spaghetti as a better pregame meal for his 280-pound linemen than the traditional lean beef. Today, just about any runner knows that spaghetti is a better premarathon meal than, say, scrambled eggs or steak, but that knowledge resulted from some pain suffered by us guinea pigs.

We now know that the preferred fuel for the endurance athlete is carbohydrate, because it is easy to digest and easy to convert into energy. Carbohydrates convert quickly into glucose (a form of sugar that circulates in the blood) and glycogen (the form of glucose stored in muscle tissue and the liver). Proteins and fats also convert into glucose/glycogen, but at a greater energy cost. The body normally can store about 2,000 calories worth of glycogen in the muscle, enough for maybe 20 miles of running.

Can better nutrition create better athletes? Ann C. Grandjean, Ed.D., director of the International Center for Sports Nutrition, frowns at the question and gives an indirect, one-word answer: "Genetics!" What she means is that great athletes are born with the ability to succeed, a gift of good genes that allows them— when properly trained and fed—to run and jump and throw faster and higher and farther than their less genetically gifted opponents. In suggesting better nutrition for long-distance runners, sports nutritionists can't promise you success—but at least you won't fail because of poor nutrition.

How important is good nutrition? Frederick C. Hagerman, Ph.D., of Ohio University, is a nutritional consultant for the Cincinnati Reds baseball team. Dr. Hagerman led off a conference in Columbus, Ohio, on "Nutrition for the Marathon and Other Endurance Sports" before the 1992 men's Olympic marathon trials by saying that the second most important question asked by athletes is, "What should I eat to make me stronger, better and faster for my sport?" (The most important question, he said, is, "How do I train?") Dr. Hagerman claims that too many athletes have no idea how to eat properly to maximize their performances.

There are three important areas of the distance runner's diet. One is overall nutrition, the ability to maintain high energy levels during training. Second is prerace nutrition, what you eat in the last few days before running to ensure a good performance. Third is what you consume (mostly liquids) during the race itself to make sure that you maximize performance—and get to the finish line on your own two feet. This chapter covers the first two, training nutrition and prerace nutrition, and your body's needs *during* the race are covered in chapter 14.

Special Needs of Runners in Training

When you run long distances, your energy requirements rise. In an article on endurance exercise in *The Physician and Sportsmedicine,* Walter R. Frontera, M.D., and Richard P. Adams, Ph.D., comment: "During sustained exercise such as marathon running, total body energy requirements increase 10 to 20 times above resting values." Runners need to eat more of the proper foods to fuel their muscles. They also need to drink more, particularly in warm weather.

At the seminar in Columbus, Linda Houtkooper, Ph.D., a registered dietitian at the University of Arizona, made clear that endurance athletes in particular should get most of their calories from carbohydrates.

No argument there. The only problem is that with 35,000 items in the supermarket, marathon runners sometimes need help determining which foods are highest in carbohydrates. Unless you plan to eat spaghetti three meals a day (and even pasta contains 13 percent protein and 4 percent fat), you may need to start reading labels.

Dr. Houtkooper explained that the body requires at least 40 nutrients that are classified into six nutritional components: proteins, carbohydrates, fats, vitamins, minerals and water. "These nutrients cannot be made in the body," says Dr. Houtkooper, "and so must be supplied from solid or liquid foods." She listed six categories that form the fundamentals of a nutritionally adequate food selection plan: fruits, vegetables, grains/legumes, lean meats, low-fat milk products and fats/sweets (in descending order of priority).

Recommendations for a healthy diet suggest 20 percent protein, 30 percent fat and 50 percent carbohydrate. But all carbohydrates aren't created alike. There are simple carbohydrates, which include sugar, honey, jam and any food such as sweets and soft drinks that get most of their calories from sugar; nutritionists recommend that these simple carbos make up only 10 percent of your diet. It's complex carbohydrates you should concentrate on: the starch in plant foods, which include fruits, vegetables, bread, pasta and legumes.

Endurance athletes particularly benefit from fuel-efficient complex carbohydrates because of the extra calories we burn each day. We need to aim for even more total carbohydrates than the suggested 50 percent. We can eat (in fact, may *need* to eat) more total calories without worrying about weight gain. High-mileage athletes may want to supplement their diets with high-carbohydrate drinks to ensure sufficient energy for their daily long runs. We can also afford a somewhat higher ratio of simple vs. complex carbohydrates in our diets—although some nutritionists might argue with me on this point.

You don't need to patronize Italian restaurants to ensure an adequate supply of complex carbohydrates (although runners attending the Boston Marathon usually head to the North End, an Italian neighborhood with many excellent restaurants). I sometimes choose a Chinese restaurant, because rice is also high in carbohydrates. And Nancy Clark, R.D., director of nutrition services for SportsMedicine Brookline in Boston, Massachusetts, and author of *Nancy Clark's Sports Nutrition Guidebook* (among the best books on the subject) points out that you can get plenty of carbos in most American restaurants. If you eat soup (such as minestrone, bean, rice or noodle), potatoes, breads and vegetables along with your main dish, and maybe grab a piece of apple cobbler off the dessert tray, you can end up eating more carbohydrates than fats or protein. (For a list of good high-carbohydrate choices, see "High-Carbohydrate Foods" on page 114.)

Checking Out Your Diet

I don't spend a lot of time agonizing over what I eat, but the last time a dietitian evaluated my diet, I averaged 12 percent protein, 19 percent fat and 69 percent carbohydrate over a typical three-day period. Fifty-two percent of total calories was complex carbohydrates and 16 percent was simple carbohydrates.

The nutritional analysis of my diet also showed I was getting more than the recommended daily allowances of vitamins and minerals, so I don't take supplements. And my cholesterol count usually hovers within a few points of 185, with a favorable HDL ratio. If I have succeeded with my dietary goals, I believe it to be for two reasons.

A healthy breakfast. You can think of a good breakfast as a fast start out of the blocks. Each morning, I drink two or three eight-ounce glasses of orange juice and usually eat a high-fiber breakfast cereal with skim milk, piled high with raisins, bananas and whatever other fruits are in season: strawberries, raspberries, blueberries. A couple of times when we were out of milk, I substituted orange juice on my cereal. Yes, it sounds disgusting, but don't knock it until you've tried it.

I also eat two slices of toast spread with margarine or butter. Two days a week, I'll eat a soft-boiled egg. Sometimes on Sundays between my long run and church, my wife and I will treat ourselves to a special breakfast with coffee cake (or pancakes, waffles or French toast), bacon and scrambled eggs with mozzarella cheese.

Joanne Milkereit's refrigerator. Okay, this needs some explaining. Joanne Milkereit was the chief nutritionist at the Hyde Park Co-op, an upscale grocery store near the University of Chicago, when we collaborated to write the *Runner's Cookbook* back in 1979. (She now works as a consulting nutri-

High-Carbohydrate Foods

The traditional prerace meal for marathoners is spaghetti. With a wife of Italian origin, I also reap the culinary benefits of a tradition that literally demands frequent doses of pasta. But spaghetti (or macaroni or other forms of pasta) every day can become boring, particularly when you're trying to carbo-load the week before a marathon. Fortunately, there are many foods you can eat that will guarantee that your diet is high in carbohydrates both during training and before races.

In *Nancy Clark's Sports Nutrition Guidebook*, the author, a dietitian, lists the following carbohydrate-rich foods.

Fruits	**Vegetables**	**Grains, Legumes and Potatoes**
Apples	Broccoli	
Apricots, dried	Carrots	Baked beans
Bananas	Corn	Lentils
Fruit Roll-Ups	Green beans	Potato, baked
Oranges	Peas	Rice
Raisins	Tomato sauce	Spaghetti
	Winter squash	Stuffing
	Zucchini	

tionist at the Medical University of South Carolina.)

While we were working on the cookbook, Milkereit told me that every runner should tape the following words on his or her refrigerator: *Eat a wide variety of lightly processed foods.*

Go back and reread this phrase. Think about it. By *wide variety,* she means you sample all the food groups. When foods are *lightly processed,* you don't destroy all the vitamins.

What does she mean by *lightly processed?* Beware of foods that come wrapped in plastic or that you can buy at a fast food restaurant—although several restaurants have started to offer such fare as low-fat burgers, carrot sticks and nutritious salads. Another food rule comes from Pete Pfitzinger, a 1984 and 1988 Olympic marathoner. He once told me, "I don't put anything in my mouth that's been invented in the last 25 years." That may

Breads, Rolls and Crackers
Bagel
Bran muffin
English muffin
Graham crackers
Matzo
Pancakes
Pita bread
Saltines
Submarine roll
Waffles
Whole-grain bread

Breakfast Cereals
Cream of Wheat
Granola, low-fat varieties
Grape-Nuts
Muesli
Oatmeal
Raisin Bran

Beverages
Apple juice
Apricot nectar
Cola drinks

Cran-raspberry juice
Orange juice

Sweets, Snacks and Desserts
Cranberry sauce
Fig bars
Fruit yogurt
Honey
Maple syrup
Pop-Tarts
Strawberry jam

Clark also warns that some foods that runners assume are high in carbohydrates may have many of their calories hidden in fat. These foods include croissants, Ritz crackers, thin-crust pizza (as opposed to thick-crust) and granola. When in doubt, Clark advises, read labels.

be a bit too extreme, but if you pay attention to these two messages, you probably can't go wrong with your diet.

Judy Tillapaugh, R.D., of Fort Wayne, Indiana, believes that while runners understand the value of carbo-loading before a marathon, they don't give equal attention to day-to-day meal plans. "Endurance athletes need to continually replace energy stores with a diet high in carbohydrates, low in fat and with enough protein to maintain muscle," says Tillapaugh. "Some weight-conscious runners don't eat enough."

And you need to spread your calories throughout the day by snacking, choosing healthy fare such as fruit, graham crackers, yogurt or bagels. If you need 3,500 calories daily, you can't pack them into one or two meals. Athletes often neglect breakfast, then wonder why they're tired while running in the evening.

Does a good diet mean no treats? My measured intake of 16 percent of calories from simple carbohydrates might be considered high for "healthy" people, but not necessarily for a competitive athlete. "Athletes are told to avoid junk foods," says Dr. Grandjean, "but the reality is that if you are eating 4,000 calories a day, once you have taken in those first 2,000 calories—assuming you've done a reasonably intelligent job of selecting foods—you've probably obtained all the nutrients you need. You don't need to worry about vitamins and minerals, because you've already supplied your needs. You can afford foods high in sugar, so-called 'empty calories,' because you need energy. Your problem sometimes is finding enough time to eat."

Sports nutrition thus comes down to a management problem.

Distance Runners *Need* Calories

The importance of general nutrition—as opposed to prerace nutrition—is that you need adequate energy for training. And unlike the general population, you may need to eat more to help maintain your weight. If you're a 150-pound person running 50 miles a week to prepare for a marathon, you need approximately 5,000 calories a week more than a sedentary person, and most of those calories should come from carbohydrates. Since carbohydrates are bulkier than fats or protein, the sheer volume of food high-mileage runners must eat can become a problem.

Dr. Grandjean says that among the athletes she advises, distance runners are most knowledgeable about nutrition because their energy needs are so high. And those most talented, the ones already on top, often have the best nutrition. Fred Brouns of the Nutrition Research Center at the University of Limburg in the Netherlands studied cyclists competing in the Tour de France, both in the laboratory and during the race. Brouns discovered that those finishing near the front were those who were most successful at managing their diets. "Endurance athletes must pay close attention to food intake if they expect to keep energy levels high," says Brouns.

In the Tour, cyclists frequently burn *5,000 calories a day!* There's no way Tour competitors can ride five or six hours a day and have time to eat that much, so they take much of their calories in liquid form while riding. Although most runners don't have anywhere near the energy requirements of a Tour cyclist, some high-mileage runners like to use high-carbohydrate drinks as a dietary supplement.

Nancy Ditz, the top U.S. finisher at the 1987 world championship and 1988 Olympic marathons, took an intelligent approach to diet. Between those two marathons, Ditz decided she wanted to leave nothing to chance when it came to race preparation. Following the suggestion of her coach, Rod Dixon, she sought nutritional advice.

Ditz didn't go to a standard dietitian but spoke with Jerry Attaway, an assistant coach with the San Francisco 49ers. Attaway manages that highly successful team's strength training, rehabilitation and diet programs. Attaway determined that, based on her energy expenditure while training 100 miles a week, Ditz needed an even higher percentage of carbohydrates than she was getting.

"Even though I was eating a pretty good diet, my carbohydrate intake still wasn't enough," Ditz recalls. She started using Exceed, a high-carbohydrate drink. (Such drinks are most effective immediately after exercise, when they can be most quickly absorbed.) Her calcium intake needed to be higher, so she also started drinking buttermilk with meals.

Ditz feared Attaway might ask her to cut out one of her favorite treats—cinnamon rolls at breakfast—but instead he eliminated mayonnaise on her sandwich at lunch. "That was a minor behavioral change for a major change in my ratio of fat to carbohydrate," she says. (In two tablespoons of mayonnaise, you get 202 calories that are 100 percent fat!)

Ditz explained that Attaway identified foods that did the most damage to her diet, then asked, "Which do you *really* like?" He let her keep those, then eliminated the rest.

Ideally, long-distance runners interested in maximizing their performances in the marathon should find someone as knowledgeable as Jerry Attaway to tell them how to eat. If I had to offer a single piece of dietary advice to every person who reads this book—regardless of whether or not you have Olympian aspirations—it would be to consult a dietitian. (The American Dietetic Association's referral network at 1-800-366-1655 can help you find a sports nutritionist.) Have that dietitian analyze your diet and recommend what to eat and what not to eat. Then follow that advice.

Eating before the Race

Pasta has become the de rigueur prerace feast for marathoners. No major marathon is without its night-before spaghetti dinner, which has assumed almost ceremonial aspects.

The spaghetti dinner, of course, has more than a ceremonial purpose. In eating high-carbohydrate pasta, we want to make sure our bodies have adequate glycogen, the fuel supply stored in the muscles that allows the most efficient form of energy metabolism. The more glycogen you can store, the faster you can run for longer periods of time, because when muscle glycogen is depleted, muscles contract poorly. But a well-fueled athlete also needs a full supply of glycogen for the liver, a "processing station" that sends fuel through the bloodstream to the muscles. So in addition to having your fuel tank full, you also need a full carburetor.

Various diets have been devised in attempts to ensure maximum glycogen storage. Carbohydrate loading—which involves depletion and replenishment—became popular in the mid-1970s following research in Scandinavia. The regimen began with a 20-mile run to exhaustion one week before the marathon to deplete muscles of all available glycogen. For three days following that purge, the athlete followed a high-protein, low-carbohydrate diet designed to keep glycogen stores artificially low. Midweek, the athlete switched to a low-protein, high-carbohydrate diet to overload the muscles with glycogen during the final three days before the race. The theory was if you deplete yourself of glycogen, you would absorb more when you did eat carbohydrates—like a sponge that, squeezed dry, absorbs more water than a damp one.

Carbo-loading seemed to work with marathoners—at least sometimes. I experimented with it and had both good and bad results. (One problem scientists have in measuring anything as complicated as effect of diet on performance is that so many other variables are present.)

Most experts today believe that runners should avoid the carbo-loading featuring depletion and replenishment. The problem is the depletion part of the cycle, the 20-miler one week before the marathon. Enlightened coaches say that 20 miles is too long and hard a run so close to a marathon. They recommend more than a week-long taper, which wouldn't allow any depletion runs. Also, the high-protein diet three days following the depletion run was so severe that runners often became depressed while following it. I certainly did. Eating became no fun—and as an upbeat psychological mood may be as important to performance as glycogen stores, the depletion phase soon lost favor.

And later research by Dr. Costill at Ball State University suggested that the depletion phase was unnecessary because you could achieve equally high glycogen levels with only the three-day high-carbohydrate phase. Most of us shouted "Hallelujah" and never went back.

So the current advice is to concentrate heavily on eating carbohydrates those final days before the marathon. When someone says "carbo-loading" today, that's usually what they mean, not the seven-day depletion/replenishment cycle. For someone like me, used to following a high-carbo diet, this requires only a few changes in the regular daily routine. This is good, because you don't want to subject your system to any radically different changes just before you're about to run 26 miles.

If you're racing out of town, you may even want to take along some snacks to eat between the pasta dinner and the race the next morning. Dried fruits can be particularly useful, especially if you're competing in a foreign country where you're not used to the food.

Last-Minute Loading

Carbo-loading shouldn't stop with the pasta dinner; scientists tell us it should continue on the starting line to ensure maximum prerace nutrition. W. Michael Sherman, Ph.D., of Ohio State University, tested trained cyclists pedaling indoors, feeding them five grams of carbohydrate per kilogram of body weight three hours before exercise. Both power and endurance increased when athletes ate before exercise. (For a 165-pound cyclist, that would be about the amount of carbohydrate in 12 bagels or 7 baked potatoes.) Dr. Sherman explains: "The cyclists were able to maintain a higher output for a longer period of time before fatiguing."

Other studies have shown improved performance four hours after eating. "We can safely say that if you have a carbohydrate feeding three to four hours before a marathon, you can enhance performance," says Dr. Sherman.

Admittedly, marathoners tolerate solids in their stomachs less well than cyclists. Dr. Sherman suggests runners either delay eating their prerace pasta until late evening or rise early for a high-carbohydrate breakfast such as pancakes or toast and orange juice. Liquid meals featuring high-carbohydrate drinks may work best for races near dawn. Dr. Sherman warns, however, that runners try this first in practice or before minor races.

In fact, practice may let you adjust to a different type of prerace nutrition than you thought possible, including solid food an hour before the race. "You can train your body to do almost anything," says Tillapaugh, who says her favorite snack before races is a bagel or low-fat crackers.

Doug Kurtis, the multimarathon runner from Michigan, however, usually eats his last meal the night before. "Rarely will I eat anything the morning of a race," he says, "unless there's a late start, such as noon at Boston. I'd rather lie in bed an extra hour than get up just to eat. Some runners can eat and be ready to run an hour later, but I find I need three to four hours to digest my food before I feel comfortable running. I've experimented with eating two to three hours before, but it just didn't work."

"The main thing is not to do anything out of the ordinary," says Ed Eyestone, a 1988 and 1992 Olympic marathoner. "Yet, you have to be flexible enough to go with the flow and eat what's available. If you're programmed to eat pancakes precisely seven hours before a marathon, you may be disappointed."

Experience has taught me that eating as close to three hours before a race gives my stomach sufficient time to digest the food and allow me to clear my intestines without fear of having to duck into the bushes at the five-mile mark. Closer than that, however, and I'm asking for trouble. This can be a problem if you're running a race like the Honolulu Marathon with its predawn start. But I've gotten up as early as 2:30 A.M. to eat breakfast before that race, and I notice I'm not always alone in the hotel coffee shop.

I'll order orange juice, toast or maybe a Danish roll and/or some applesauce along with a single cup of coffee. Some experts warn against coffee, because it's a diuretic, but it helps clear my bowels. If you're running an international race—and I've run marathons in Berlin, Athens, Rome and other major cities—you may not be able to get a typical American breakfast, but the continental breakfast of coffee and rolls (with or without jelly) works quite well.

If the coffee shop doesn't open early enough, those snacks in the suitcase may come in handy. I'm less fussy. Practically every hotel has a soft drink machine on each floor, and frequently a can of pop is my last meal before a morning marathon.

I'll stop drinking two hours before the race, as it takes approximately that long for liquids to migrate from your mouth to your bladder. Another one to two cups just before the start will help you tank up for the race, and this liquid will most likely be utilized before it reaches your bladder. If you drink much in that two-hour period, however, you may find yourself worrying about how you will relieve yourself several miles into the race. Following his bronze-medal performance at the 1991 World Championships, Steve Spence told *Runner's World* that he drank so much that he had to urinate three times during the race without breaking stride. Personally, I'd prefer to avoid that.

CHAPTER 12

Predicting Pace and
PERFORMANCE

L et's talk about predicting performance. How do you pick the pace
that's right for you? How can you anticipate a reasonable finishing time?

Unless you have some idea of what you're capable of, you
won't know how fast you should be running each mile. Run too
slowly at the start, and you may find yourself too fresh at the
end with a slower finishing time than you had anticipated.
That's all right if you're a first-timer intent only on finishing, but
not if you're a seasoned runner hoping to improve. Start too
quickly, of course, and you risk hitting the Wall.

If you chart your times during workouts—speed workouts as
well as your long runs—you probably have an approximate idea
of how fast you can run. Your times in preliminary races also can
give you a clue. But there are more precise ways to predict performance in a marathon and also more precise ways to determine how fast you should run each mile.

Measuring Human Performance

With increased interest in fitness sports during the last quarter century, there has been a simultaneous rise in the number of
laboratories dedicated to measuring human performance.
Scientists have become interested in why some athletes outper-
form others.

The most common measuring device in any running-oriented

human performance laboratory is the treadmill, a moving belt where you can run in place while various measurements are made. The most common measurement is maximum VO_2, the volume of oxygen a person can consume during exercise. This relates both to the heart's capacity for pumping oxygen-rich blood to the muscles and how efficiently those muscles extract and utilize that oxygen.

Maximum VO_2, often referred to simply as VO_2 max, is calculated from the number of milliliters of oxygen your body can absorb during 60 seconds, per kilogram of body weight. VO_2 max is measured in milliliters of oxygen per kilogram of body weight per minute (ml/kg/mn). Within certain limits, the higher your VO_2 max, the better your ability to perform. A talented runner with a VO_2 max of 70 could be expected to run a 10-K in around 31 minutes and a marathon in 2:23. An average runner, say someone with the ability to run a 10-K in about 45 minutes, probably has a VO_2 max around 45. Untrained or sedentary individuals would have still lower levels.

But other factors affect performance. One is running technique, or efficiency, what exercise scientists often refer to as "economy." Runners succeed only partly because of superior cardiovascular systems. You only need see the people near the front of the pack to understand that. Most are smooth, efficient runners who waste little energy covering the ground. An economical runner might run a marathon 10 or 20 minutes faster than someone with an equal VO_2 max who is a less efficient runner.

In general, however, if you know your VO_2 max, you can predict your performance. If you can *improve* your VO_2 max, you may be able to improve your performance.

Oxygen Power

Alas, not everybody has the opportunity to determine their VO_2 max. Most human performance laboratories are geared to doing research, not testing joggers for their own information. Most medical centers do what are known as "symptom-limited" exercise stress tests to diagnose heart conditions, but they usually stop short of VO_2 max. They don't—and usually *won't*—measure it. So how does the average runner determine his or her VO_2 max?

Jack Daniels, Ph.D., exercise physiologist at the State University of New York in Cortland and coach of that school's cross-country team, has developed oxygen power tables to help predict performance. Dr. Daniels, formerly a top-ranked pentathlete, is among America's most respected sports scientists. He has also worked as a coach adviser to top athletes such as Jim Ryun, Alberto Salazar and Joan Benoit Samuelson. For several years, Dr. Daniels worked in Eugene, Oregon, for Athletics West, Nike's sponsored team.

Dr. Daniels developed his oxygen power tables in collaboration with Jimmy Gilbert, one of his former runners and a programmer for NASA in Houston. By doing treadmill and track measurements on runners of various abilities (and collecting available data on others), Dr. Daniels and Gilbert were able to relate VO_2 max scores to performances. The two researchers developed a set of tables, which they published in a book titled *Oxygen Power*. (Copies of the book can be obtained from Dr. Daniels at Box 5062, Cortland, NY 13045.) Using these tables, a runner can use any recent performance to predict something called *VDOT*. This value combines VO_2 max with running economy into a single value that *approximates* VO_2 max. The VDOT can be used to predict with some accuracy how fast you can run at distances from 800 meters to 50-K. A runner can also equate performance at one distance to a performance at another. For instance, if you have the ability to run 40 minutes for a 10-K, you can probably (assuming proper training) run near three hours for the marathon.

If you know how fast you run a 10-K, or any other distance, you can predict your VDOT. If you run a 10-K in 49:00, you probably have a VDOT of 41.0. If you improve your time to 48:30, it's probably because your VDOT also has improved, to 41.5.

Beginning on page 126 is an adapted and condensed version of the Daniels oxygen power tables for five commonly run distances: the mile, 5-K (3.1 miles), 10-K (6.2 miles), half-marathon (13.1 miles) and marathon (42.2-K or 26.2 miles). This oxygen power table includes 65 different levels, showing VDOT values that might be achieved by runners at various levels, from a beginning jogger to a world-class athlete. The first level (VDOT 30) shows someone capable of running 63:46 for a 10-K. The final level describes performances for better than the current world records.

How to Use the Table

You should not attempt to measure your ability using the oxygen power table if you are a beginning runner. You need to condition your body before you test your abilities.

If you are reasonably well conditioned, have been training for several months and have no serious medical conditions (as determined by an exercise stress test) that would prevent you from running as hard and as fast as you can, you are ready to test your oxygen power.

The basic test distance is one mile, although seasoned runners may prefer 10-K, the most common competitive race distance. To test yourself over one mile, you can go to a nearby athletic facility that has a 400-meter track and time yourself for four laps with a stopwatch. (Since a mile is slightly longer than 1600 meters, you may want to make adjustments by either running the additional ten-yard difference between 1600 meters and one mile, or adding several seconds to your time.)

If you are an experienced runner, you may prefer to test your VO_2 max in a race, possibly at the 10-K distance. It can be easier to push yourself to maximum performance while running in the company of others. If you go this route, be certain that the race organizers have accurately measured the course. Choose a race where the course is certified by the TAC/RRCA certification committee. Most better races note their certification on the entry blank.

To get a more accurate idea of your level, you may decide to test yourself over a series of distances, adding half-marathon or marathon times. Don't be surprised, however, if the chart indicated a higher VDOT for your speed at some distances than others. If you have more fast-twitch muscles (for short, explosive effort) than slow-twitch muscles (for sustained effort), you're more likely to run the mile fast than the marathon. If the reverse is true, your marathon time may be best. Your level of conditioning also may affect your ability to perform at the longer distances. Obviously, the best predictor of your marathon perfor-

(continued on page 128)

Oxygen Power Table

VDOT	Mile	5000 Meters	10-K	Half-Marathon	Marathon
30	9:11	30:40	63:46	2:21:04	4:49:17
31	8:55	29:51	62:03	2:17:21	4:41:57
32	8:41	29:05	60:26	2:13:49	4:34:59
33	8:27	28:21	58:54	2:10:27	4:28:22
34	8:14	27:39	57:26	2:07:16	4:22:03
35	8:01	27:00	56:03	2:04:13	4:16:03
36	7:49	26:22	54:44	2:01:19	4:10:19
37	7:38	25:46	53:29	1:58:34	4:04:50
38	7:27	25:12	52:17	1:55:55	3:59:35
39	7:17	24:39	51:09	1:53:24	3:54:34
40	7:07	24:08	50:03	1:50:59	3:49:45
41	6:58	23:38	49:01	1:48:40	3:45:09
42	6:49	23:09	48:01	1:46:27	3:40:43
43	6:41	22:41	47:04	1:44:20	3:36:28
44	6:32	22:15	46:09	1:42:17	3:32:23
45	6:25	21:50	45:16	1:40:20	3:28:26
46	6:17	21:25	44:25	1:38:27	3:24:39
47	6:10	21:02	43:36	1:36:38	3:21:00
48	6:03	20:39	42:50	1:34:53	3:17:29
49	5:56	20:18	42:04	1:33:12	3:14:06
50	5:50	19:57	41:21	1:31:35	3:10:49
51	5:44	19:36	40:39	1:30:02	3:07:39
52	5:38	19:17	39:59	1:28:31	3:04:36
53	5:32	18:58	39:20	1:27:04	3:01:39
54	5:27	18:40	38:42	1:25:40	2:58:47
55	5:21	18:22	38:06	1:24:18	2:56:01
56	5:16	18:05	37:31	1:23:00	2:53:20
57	5:11	17:49	36:57	1:21:43	2:50:45
58	5:06	17:33	36:24	1:20:30	2:48:14
59	5:02	17:17	35:52	1:19:18	2:45:47
60	4:57	17:03	35:22	1:18:09	2:43:25
61	4:53	16:48	34:52	1:17:02	2:41:08
62	4:49	16:34	34:23	1:15:57	2:38:54

VDOT	Mile	5000 Meters	10-K	Half-Marathon	Marathon
63	4:45	16:20	33:55	1:14:54	2:36:44
64	4:41	16:07	33:28	1:13:53	2:34:38
65	4:37	15:54	33:01	1:12:53	2:32:35
66	4:33	15:42	32:35	1:11:56	2:30:36
67	4:30	15:29	32:11	1:11:00	2:28:40
68	4:26	15:18	31:46	1:10:05	2:26:47
69	4:23	15:06	31:23	1:09:12	2:24:57
70	4:19	14:55	31:00	1:08:21	2:23:10
71	4:16	14:44	30:38	1:07:31	2:21:26
72	4:13	14:33	30:16	1:06:42	2:19:44
73	4:10	14:23	29:55	1:05:54	2:18:05
74	4:07	14:13	29:34	1:05:08	2:16:29
75	4:04	14:03	29:14	1:04:23	2:14:55
76	4:02	13:54	28:55	1:03:39	2:13:23
76.5	4:00.2	13:49	28:45	1:03:18	2:12:38
77	3:58.8	13:44	28:36	1:02:56	2:11:54
77.5	3:57.5	13:40	28:26	1:02:35	2:11:10
78	3:56.2	13:35	28:17	1:02:15	2:10:27
78.5	3:54.9	13:31	28:08	1:01:54	2:09:44
79	3:53.7	13:26	27:59	1:01:34	2:09:02
79.5	3:52.4	13:22.1	27:49.9	1:01:14	2:08:20
80	3:51.2	13:17.8	27:41.2	1:00:54	2:07:38
80.5	3:49.9	13:13.5	27:32.5	1:00:34.9	2:26:57.5
81	3:48.7	13:09.3	27:23.9	1:00:15.6	2:06:17.1
81.5	3:47.5	13:05.2	27:15.4	59:56.6	2:05:37.2
82	3:46.4	13:01.1	27:07.1	59:37.9	2:04:57.8
82.5	3:45.2	12:57.0	26:58.8	59:19.3	2:04:18.8
83	3:44.1	12:53.0	26:50.6	59:01.0	2:03:40.3
83.5	3:42.9	12:49.1	26:42.5	58:42.9	2:03:02.2
84	3:41.8	12:45.2	26:34.6	58:25.0	2:02:24.5
84.5	3:40.7	12:41.3	26:26.7	58:07.3	2:01:47.3
85	3:39.6	12:37.5	26:18.9	57:49.8	2:01:10.5

mance will be a VDOT level based on longer distances rather than shorter.

When you have completed your test run, whether on a track or the road, look at the table and find the number closest to the time you ran. Locate the corresponding VDOT, which is your approximate VO_2 max. The table will also tell you how fast you might run at other race distances—assuming you train properly for those distances.

Having established your oxygen power level, you now can use that level as a guide to predicting your theoretical race pace.

How accurate are the Daniels and Gilbert numbers? From a theoretical standpoint, they're *very* accurate. From a realistic standpoint, however, they're flawed, because people with lower VO_2 maxes may have trouble meeting the times predicted for all distances. A person who jogs a mile in 9 or 10 minutes may have trouble finishing a 10-K, much less running it in nearly 60 minutes. And running a marathon in anything under five hours may be out of the question—at least until he or she has trained for that distance.

In general, the better trained you are as a runner, the more accurate you're liable to find the Daniels and Gilbert numbers.

A Second Opinion

Here's another method of predicting performance. These figures come from George Myers of St. Joseph, Michigan, an engineer with the Whirlpool Corporation in Benton Harbor. He has an extensive sports background. While attending Iowa State University, he placed second in the 1952 NCAA (National Collegiate Athletic Association) wrestling championships and later took up bicycle touring, marathons and triathlons. Myers has too much upper-body mass to have great success as a runner. But he loves to run and also enjoys playing with numbers. After participating in about 150 races (including 20 marathons) and talking with coaches and other runners, Myers decided to develop his own race prediction table, based more on experience than on scientific research.

Myers contends that not all runners slow their pace as much from the 10-K to the marathon. "Fast runners slow down less than slower runners," he contends. While the pace of a fast runner capable of 30:00 for a 10-K might slow by 10 percent to 2:19:15 for the marathon, he projects that a runner capable of 40:00 for a 10-K will run the marathon in 3:09:53, a slowdown of 12.5 percent.

"Runners do slow down on a straight line or linear basis from the 10-K to the marathon," says Myers, "but this is true only if the runner is conditioned to run the given distance. A 40-minute 10-K runner cannot run 3:10 for the marathon unless he trains for that distance."

The prediction times in Myers's table assume a fast course, good weather and a well-prepared and rested runner.

Myers Performance Prediction Table

5-K	10-K	15-K	20-K	Half-Marathon	25-K	Marathon
13:40	28:00	42:37	57:39	1:01:00	1:13:06	2:09:22
14:38	30:00	45:42	1:01:52	1:05:28	1:18:30	2:19:15
15:37	32:00	48:47	1:06:05	1:09:57	1:23:55	2:29:12
16:35	34:00	51:52	1:10:19	1:14:27	1:29:21	2:39:15
17:34	36:00	54:58	1:14:34	1:18:58	1:34:49	2:49:22
18:32	38:00	58:04	1:18:50	1:23:29	1:40:19	2:59:35
19:31	40:00	1:01:10	1:23:06	1:28:02	1:45:49	3:09:53
20:29	42:00	1:04:16	1:27:24	1:32:35	1:51:22	3:20:15
21:28	44:00	1:07:23	1:31:41	1:37:09	1:56:55	3:30:43
22:26	46:00	1:10:30	1:36:00	1:41:44	2:02:30	3:41:16
23:25	48:00	1:13:37	1:40:19	1:46:20	2:08:06	3:51:54
24:23	50:00	1:16:45	1:44:40	1:50:56	2:13:44	4:02:37
25:22	52:00	1:19:53	1:49:00	1:55:34	2:19:23	4:13:25
26:20	54:00	1:23:01	1:53:22	2:00:13	2:25:04	4:24:19

Still More Predictors

Let me offer you a simpler method of using your 10-K time to predict marathon performance, one suggested by Melvin H. Williams, Ph.D., of Old Dominion University in Norfolk, Virginia. Dr. Williams suggests multiplying your 10-K time by 4.66. According to this theory, a runner capable of 36:00 for a 10-K should be able to run a 2:47:45 marathon. The Daniels and Gilbert table would predict 2:46:15; Myers would suggest

2:49:22. David Cowein, a coach from Morrilton, Arkansas, suggests a simpler strategy of multiplying 10-K time by 5, which results in an even more conservative prediction of 3:00:00. If space were available, I could offer you a half dozen other tables developed by knowledgeable individuals. One I use most often myself is in the book *Computerized Running Programs,* written by James B. Gardner and J. Gerry Purdy in 1970 and still available from *Track & Field News* (2570 El Camino Real, Suite 606, Los Altos, CA 94040). Gardner and Purdy claim a 36:09 10-K predicts a 2:49:38 for the marathon.

Outsmarting the Boston Course

In 1964, before my best time at Boston, I determined my pace strategy by consulting back editions of newspapers to determine the splits at various points for runners who had run times near the time I hoped to achieve. Today's runners, used to having each mile clearly marked often with digital display clocks, may find it difficult to believe that Boston's organizers *never* offered split times, which would have been meaningless since the checkpoints were all at odd distances, such as 6½ miles.

Nevertheless, the Boston papers usually published those splits of the leaders at these odd distances, and by visiting the public library and examining back copies, I carefully constructed a pace chart for a 2:21 finish. Before the race, I wrote my splits on the back of my hand with ballpoint pen. (Following the race, one of the reporters referred to me as "the methodical Higdon" for doing this.) My plans went out the window somewhat when I decided to stay with the front runners, and I held the lead for several miles leading into the hills around 17 or 18 miles. After losing several places, I closed strong in the final miles.

Here are my predicted and actual paces, with an *e* for times I estimated.

So what method should you use? There's no concrete answer. If you're a highly talented and well-trained runner who runs fast, you probably will find the Daniels and Gilbert table most accurate; if you are less gifted and with less time to train, you may prefer one of the more conservative charts. Achieving success as a long-distance runner remains as much an art as a science. You need to apply both art and science if you expect to succeed.

Cowein also warns that you should pick a realistic goal: "No matter how well you feel on race day, if you're a 3:00 marathoner, you're not going to run 2:30. Be honest with yourself."

Checkpoint	Mile	Predicted	Actual
Framingham	6.5	34:30	34:10
Natick	10.5	54:30	53:50
Wellesley	13.5	1:10:00	1:09:00
Auburndale	17.5	1:54:00	1:55(e)
Heartbreak	21.5	2:08:00	2:09(e)
Finish	26.2	2:21:00	2:21:55

You can see that I did a respectable job of predicting performance, particularly when you consider that my marathon PR at that time was 2:36:13 at Boston the previous year. But after a successful track career, I was just beginning to learn the secrets of long-distance running and had won the National Amateur Athletic Union 30-K championships the month before.

Runners who challenge Boston today have an easier task, not only because there are markers every mile, but also because at the prerace Expo they can get a computer printout with any pace they desire designed to match the course topography. (This service is available at many of the largest marathons.)

The Right Pace

Once you obtain an estimate of your finishing time, you can determine the best pace to obtain that time. Again, experts differ, and there are various ways to predetermine race pace. The simplest is to run at the same speed mile after mile for the full distance.

To run a three-hour marathon, you would simply run 26 consecutive 6:52 miles. Robert Eslick, a coach from Nashville, Tennessee, claims, "All in all, I think it's no secret that even pacing works best."

Coach Tom Grogon of Cincinnati agrees: "I want my runners to run at relatively even pace. Given this, they should view those who bolt out early as foolish people whom they will catch at the end."

If you really enjoy catching people, you can try running "reverse splits." This means running the second half of the race faster than the first half. The advantage of this is that you'll be speeding up when most runners are slowing down. You'll pass others, rather than have others pass you. This can be stimulating mentally, and you'll also probably suffer less postrace muscle soreness and fatigue, because saving your fast running will let you retain your most efficient running form longer.

This strategy works best on courses with little terrain variation. Encounter a hill (uphill or down) and you may need to alter your planned pace. The Boston Marathon, for example, because of its hilly nature, keeps runners from attempting an even pace. Boston is a point-to-point course from suburban Hopkinton into the city that drops sharply in the first mile and continues downhill for most of the first 6 miles before flattening through mile 12. Then there are a series of ups and downs with the low spot on the course near 17 miles. Four hills over the next 4 miles—culminating with notorious Heartbreak Hill—slow even the best-conditioned runner. Then there's a final steady drop between miles 21 and 26. The course will defy most pace charts.

But George Myers, my engineer/analyst friend from St. Joseph, Michigan, also has studied marathon pace from the point of view of the slower runner. He determined that most runners should allow a slowdown toward the end of the race.

Myers got the idea for creating a pacing table from one designed by Joe Henderson, a senior writer for *Runner's World.* Henderson contended that most published marathon pacing guides incorrectly assumed people could run all 26 miles (not to mention the final 385 yards) at an even pace. Few runners can do that, so he developed a table based on the more common pattern of a slow beginning, a fast middle and a sag at the end.

Even world-class runners slow down in the last six miles, as their core temperatures rise (even in relatively cool weather) and their bodies perform less efficiently. In Frank Shorter's gold-medal marathon at the 1972 Olympics in Munich, his average pace in five-mile segments was 5:03.6, 4:52.4, 4:56.6, 5:03.2, and 5:15.2, for a final time of 2:12:20. In the closing stages, Shorter was still pulling away from the field because everybody else was slowing more than he.

Myers modified Henderson's tables for the Madison Marathon in Wisconsin in June 1979 and ran 3:19:58, slicing 23 minutes off his PR at the age of 48. After that, Myers decided to do some more fine-tuning. He began by dividing the 26.2-mile marathon race into segments. Then he decided upon how much time the runner should spend covering each segment, and stated it as a percentage. (See the table on page 134.)

We published Myers's tables in an article I wrote for *The Runner,* and after receiving feedback from additional runners, Myers modified the tables slightly. Myers encourages runners of all abilities to use his formula. He also emphasizes:

- Choose a realistic goal.
- Carry your pacing schedule with you. Carrying a predesigned pace table allows you to know how close you are to pace at every point in the race.
- Believe in your pace chart: Check each mile, making no changes in the first 20 miles (no matter how "good" you feel).
- Be prepared to make the necessary adjustments if the course is especially hilly.
- Meet intermediate time goals. This gives you confidence and causes the miles to pass faster.
- At 20, if you feel good, go for it; if not, hang in there.

Myers usually writes his pace carefully in large, clear numbers on a piece of paper, laminates the paper in plastic to protect it, then tapes it to his race number, upside down, so he can easily refer to it during the race. On several occasions, he has made pace charts for me. It's easy to flip the chart up each mile to see how close you are to predicted pace. It's certainly more efficient than writing your pace in ballpoint pen on your wrist, or on your number. Here's how it works.

The marathon is blocked into four segments, and you run each mile of the segment in a time that's a percentage of your desired finish time. (See below.) Myers's formula allows for slower running as you progress: Your early miles are done in 3.756 percent of your finish time, while the final miles are in 3.95 percent of the final time.

Sound complicated? It's easy to use. Figure your projected finish time in seconds. For three hours, this would be 10,800 seconds. To figure your pace for miles 0 to 12, multiply that 10,800 times 3.756 percent. This gives you a per-mile pace in seconds, 406, which equals a 6:46 pace.

Myers Pace Table for 3:00 Marathon

Mile	Percentage	Per-Mile Pace
0-12	3.756	6:46
12-18	3.8086	6:51
18-23	3.8725	6:58
23-26	3.950	7:07

One caveat concerning the Myers pace tables: They are designed under the assumption that the course is flat, with zero wind. If the course is hilly or windy you may need to make adjustments.

A tailwind—which every runner hopes for when racing on a point-to-point course—will make you run faster, sometimes as much as several minutes. On a loop course where the wind may hit you from different directions at different times of the race, you may need to make mental adjustments at midrace to stay on pace.

Temperature also can affect your pace. When race temperatures rise or fall much above or below your comfort level, you may need to throw your pace table away.

Any pace table—no matter how well designed—can be a trap, a series of numbers that can lure you into trying to keep up a faster pace than your capabilities that specific day. The best pace-setting device inevitably becomes your own mind. Experienced runners eventually know when to slow down and when to speed up. Experience thus becomes a major factor in marathon success as well as one of the fascinations of the race. Although ability and training certainly are major factors, the marathon definitely is a thinking person's race.

CHAPTER 13

Race-Day
LOGISTICS

A fter six months to a year of training—after the mileage buildup, the long runs, the taper, the carbo-loading—what can you expect once you arrive at the race site and head toward the starting line? Most veterans usually follow a well-rehearsed routine that makes their marathons easy. (Well, easier than they might otherwise be.)

Following are some suggestions that will make your race day easier—at least until the gun goes off.

Your "final" preparation begins just before you leave home, when you pack your bag. In this case, you need to heed one doctor's advice: George Sheehan, M.D., who virtually never leaves home without his runner's suitcase—a bag in the trunk of his car packed with gear in case he stops somewhere and wants to run. Dr. Sheehan once wrote in his local New Jersey newspaper column about the bag—then forgot it the next time he left for a ten-mile race in New York's Van Cortland Park.

"I had to borrow shoes, shorts and a shirt," Dr. Sheehan recalls. "I was completely outfitted by other runners, who fortunately hadn't forgotten their bags."

But running clothes and shoes are only the minimum essentials, whether you're heading for a workout or a race. Smart runners cram their bags with numerous other items.

A Runner's Suitcase

Here's an important tip from Doug Kurtis, the Michigan runner who has run more than 130 marathons: "Break everything in before you race: socks, shorts, singlet, shoes." Kurtis recommends doing one or two workouts in your race clothing to make certain everything fits and there are no problem areas, such as an imperfection inside a shoe that could cause a blister. That may not bother you in a 10-K, but it can draw blood and bring you to a halt in a marathon. "One good way to work out the bugs and test your equipment is to enter shorter races before the marathon," says Kurtis.

Here are some items you might want to include in your runner's suitcase.

The right shoes. The most essential item, obviously. Many runners like to take training shoes for warming up, then shift to a lighter racing pair. On rainy days, you'll want dry shoes for afterward. You may want to pack your racing shoes in your carry-on luggage. If the airline loses your bag, you can replace everything else, but not a well-broken-in pair of shoes. When en route to Ottawa, Ontario, for a cross-country ski race, the airline lost my bag with skis, poles and boots. The boots I borrowed were two sizes too big and the skis and poles were the wrong length. You can't carry a ski bag onto an airplane, but you can carry a pair of running shoes.

Shorts and singlet. Also obvious. Some people wear the race T-shirt they've been handed the night before, but, like Kurtis, I prefer to pretest everything. Do the shorts fit? Will the singlet or T-shirt chafe? (A snug shirt or a brand-new, unwashed one might.) Also bring a warm-up shirt to shed before you go to the start. You'll be most comfortable standing at the line if you wait until after warming up to change into a dry racing singlet. Pin your number on before leaving home.

Safety pins. Most races provide safety pins, but sometimes only two, and sometimes they run out. If you're like me, you'll want at least four to secure your number so it doesn't flap. A few races require two numbers. (At Twin Cities, you wear a back number identifying your age group, a nice touch.) Pins also come in handy for other things, such as securing your car keys in a pocket. I usually take along four pins linked together and fastened to a snap on the outside of my bag.

Entry blank. If you should get lost en route, would you be able to find the starting line? Are you certain what time the bus leaves for the start and when that start is? Use the time between warm-up and start to read all those directions you gathered with your number. You may learn some vital detail that will help you in the race.

Gloves and a cap. If the day is cold, you'll want these extra items. Whether or not you wear them in the race, gloves and a cap can help you stay warm before and after. A billed cap in summer will keep the sun off your face. As with other race gear, test them in practice for comfort. I have a torn and battered cotton cap so formless and ugly that I wouldn't want to be seen in it anywhere else but the starting line of a marathon. Another old road runner trick is to knot a white handkerchief at its four corners to wear on your head.

Varied-weight clothing. Don't assume the weather will be warm if the month is July or cold if it's January. If a freak cold wave or heat wave hits, can you cope with it? The Boston Marathon in April is notorious for unpredictable weather. I wear shorts and a regular race singlet if the temperature is going to be in the mid-40s. If it's much colder, I'll don Lycra tights and a long-sleeved shirt—a big improvement over the heavy, cotton turtleneck top I had to wear for warmth in the cold and rainy 1964 Boston Marathon.

Throwaway clothing. In large races where you may need to stand on the starting line for a long time, it's important to stay warm. If you can't take a friend to hand your discarded warm-up gear to at the last minute, take throwaway clothes that you won't mind having donated to the Salvation Army when you leave them behind. Garbage bags with armholes cut in them do protect against the wind but don't hold much warmth. Most marathons have trucks right at the line you can throw your gear into just before the start, but don't count on it. Particularly in crowded fields, you may have to stand a long time on the starting grid. Fortunately, most marathons today are so well organized that they start precisely on time.

Money. Of course you'll need money for your entry fee, if you

Your Checklist

When Ron Gunn and I lead runners on tours to races such as the Honolulu Marathon, we usually provide this checklist.

Carry-on Luggage
Racing shoes
Airline tickets
Passport and
  other documents
Toothbrush and
  toothpaste
Hotel and rental car
  confirmation
Event schedule and
  information
Itinerary
Toiletries
Credit cards

Travelers' checks
Camera and film
Wallet and money

Other Gear
Dress clothes
Dress shoes
Socks
Underwear
Coat
Gloves
Umbrella
Sunglasses
Sunscreen

Alarm clock
Race uniform
Race socks
Throwaway cold-
  weather gear
Rain suit
Swim suit
Gloves and hat
Safety pins
Petroleum jelly
Tape and adhesive
  bandages
Medicine
Special race drink

Have we forgotten anything? Experience will teach you how to organize your own runner's suitcase.

haven't preregistered. Cash also comes in handy after the race if a vendor is selling ice cream—or to take the subway home if you locked your keys in the car. Put a few extra dollars and some change in the bag that gets transported to the finish line just in case you need it. Is there a chance you might drop out? Tuck a $20 bill in your shorts pocket so you can take a taxi.

First-aid items. Pack these in a smaller bag: petroleum jelly, adhesive bandages, tape, sunscreen, aspirin, medication.

Combination lock. This comes in handy if there's a dressing room where you can stow your gear in a locker, although this is more common at track meets than at marathons. Many races today are so large that runners come dressed to run. A word to the wise: Don't take chances with expensive items. If your bag will be transported to the finish line for you, don't put expensive gear such as your Gore-Tex suit inside unless you can afford to lose it.

Food and drinks. Don't count on the race director providing your favorite beverage. And if you finish late, thirsty runners may have drunk everything before you. Pack snacks also for after the race.

Postrace clothing. Once you finish, you'll want to change into dry clothing, including socks. Also take a towel so you can dry off. You'll want to look and feel your best at the awards ceremony.

Plastic bag. Bags—the kind they gave you at the store when you bought your last pair of running shoes—come in handy after the race to isolate your sweaty gear from the rest of your clothing. A separate plastic bag for grimy shoes is also useful.

Notebook and pen. Record your finishing time, or splits, before you forget them.

Checklist. Have you forgotten anything? You won't know unless you also have a checklist of the above items. Experience eventually will guide you. When you determine what items work best in your runner's bag, make a checklist to make sure you don't leave home without them.

The Morning of the Race

For 5-K or 10-K races, I don't mind rising early and driving an hour or two to a race, and most runners feel the same. Not only do I want to avoid the extra expense of a hotel and meals away from home, but an overnight stay converts the race into an expedition requiring planning and commitment. Sometimes I like to just go, run and go home (unless, of course, I've won an age-group award).

But a marathon does require commitment, and because I usually run only one or two a year, I prefer to stay overnight before the race. Even though South Bend is only 45 minutes from my home in Michigan City, Indiana, I checked into a hotel the night before the Sunburst Marathon to avoid driving even that far on race morning and to allow myself an extra hour's sleep before the 6:00 start.

Even if it costs a little more, I prefer to stay as close as possible to the race's start and finish. Usually race directors select their headquarters hotel with this in mind. For point-to-point marathons, most runners stay near the finish line so they can head to their rooms quickly after finishing.

Getting Up and Going

Before Sunburst, I set my alarm for 4:45 A.M., then awoke from a sound sleep several minutes before it went off. I drank a 12-ounce can of Coke (my final carbo-load), then dressed and went out to warm up.

I often warm up early, at the hotel, for several reasons. First, going outside and testing the weather for yourself is more reliable than listening to weather reports on TV or radio. Second, a short run usually loosens my bowels; I'd rather use the toilet in my hotel room than stand in a long line for a Porta Potti. A half mile or a mile jog and walk usually accomplishes this.

Becoming toilet-trained is a necessity if you don't want to waste energy and time standing in long Porta Potti lines. If I'm driving to the start, I sometimes arrive with a nearly empty gas tank so I'll have an excuse to stop at a gas station and use the rest room. I'm adept at locating toilets away from the start that I can visit during my warm-up. Driving the final miles to the race, I keep my eyes open for a friendly McDonald's close enough to jog to but far enough so most of the other runners won't want to. That's one advantage of being a high-mileage runner: You can outrun the competition for an uncrowded toilet.

For my early morning warm-up, I don't usually wear my race clothes. After visiting the john and changing, I gather any extra gear I need—including my runner's bag, packed the night before—and head for the start.

Getting to the Start

Each race has its own protocol requiring careful attention (and some experience—yours or that of friends) if you don't want to get to the starting line too early or too late. At the Boston Marathon, runners board buses in downtown Boston at 8:00 A.M. (four hours before the noon start) for transportation to Hopkinton. After arriving near the start, they spend the next hour or two milling around the high school gym in suburban Hopkinton before being shooed to the starting line 30 to 60 minutes before the start. If the weather is cold or rainy, runners cram into the gym so tightly you can hardly move, much less find a spot to lie down. It's the least agreeable part of running Boston, but nevertheless it's part of the mystique of that race.

At Boston and most other large races, the elite runners are supplied transportation and a private dressing area near the start. It makes the final hour before the marathon much more comfortable, a necessity for someone seeking peak performance. Because race directors hope for fast times to please sponsors, they do what they can to make competition comfortable for top runners.

But most race directors provide well for all runners.During the fall of 1991, when I crammed six marathons into six weeks (starting all but one with the pack), I was struck by how well organized each race was and how well race directors provided the back of the pack with a reasonable amount of comfort.

Runners without the privileges of the elite dressing room need to organize themselves as much as possible on race day to minimize the hassle caused by being part of a 10,000-runner happening. This requires preplanning. Often you only learn how to cope with one specific marathon by running it once and returning the following year better prepared. Or you attend the race with friends who were there the year before and who can tell you what to expect.

On the Starting Line

Warming up is difficult at large races because at the time when you normally might be doing some final strides or a bit of jogging, you often need to stay in place to secure your position on the starting line. At marathons such as New York or Honolulu, runners are marched to the line well before the gun. It's the only way to handle the crowds of starters, but if you like to follow a particular warm-up routine as I do, it can wreak havoc with your preparation. The fortunate thing about marathons is that—unless you're an elite runner planning a 4:30 first mile—you probably don't need as much warm-up as you might for a 10-K race where you need to run fast from the gun. You may lose a minute or two with a slow start, but this may not be that important over the length of a marathon. However, the inconvenience of crowds is one reason why you may want to try a small, intimate marathon when you try for a new personal record.

At races where I plan to try for first in my age group, I position myself as close to the starting line as I can without blocking faster runners. I don't like being passed and I don't like having to pass others. It always irritates me when I see novice runners or young children lined up in the front row, where they risk being trampled once the gun sounds. How do you politely tell a novice runner who's in the wrong spot to move to the back without seeming arrogant? Usually I shrug and hope they learn before they race again. One year, after getting boxed by crowds the race organizers had failed to control at the start of the Shamrock Shuffle in Chicago, I found myself having to dodge around one runner jogging with his dog, for Pete's sake! He either started in or near the front row, or jumped in from a side street.

CHAPTER 14

Liquid Refreshment,
TO SURVIVE
AND EXCEL

I plotted my campaign with the care of Montgomery mounting an attack against Rommel. When you go out in the noonday sun—at war or in marathons—you first secure your supply lines.

At 3 miles, I found a water fountain beside the tennis courts. For relief at mile 5, I asked Bill Barkow, a fellow member of the Dunes Running Club, to turn on his front yard hose. At mile 6, I stationed Mark McGrath, a two-miler on my track team, with a jug of Gatorade. At mile 10, near the turnaround in Beverly Shores, there was a parking lot with a drinking fountain. At mile 12, massage therapist Patty Longnecker promised to turn on her sprinkler.

On the return, we'd pass McGrath, Barkow and the tennis courts again for even more fluids.

Our marathon class was running a 20-miler three weeks before the Sunburst Marathon, and it would test not only our ability to run that far but also our ability to drink enough to keep cool. Overheating can slow you down. If the weather is hot and humid enough, it can kill you. So you drink. And drink.

Survival is merely one reason why runners need to drink when they run far. The other reason is to replace lost energy and to enhance performance.

A generation ago, runners ignored fluids while running marathons because of a combination of arrogance, ignorance and a lack of aid stations. Emil Zatopek won the 1952 Olympic marathon without taking a sip. Zatopek was a track world record holder running his first 26-miler and probably didn't know how to drink on the run. He was his era's best distance runner and succeeded on talent, training and toughness.

But Zatopek's time was 2:23:03, a performance so ordinary by today's standards that it would barely get him in the top 100 in most major races—and wouldn't qualify him for the U.S. Olympic trials. The world record for women is now several minutes faster than Zatopek's best, which seems astounding to those of us old enough to remember how the gritty Czech totally dominated his competition.

Today's runners know how to drink.

They drink often: water as well as replacement fluids such as Gatorade, Exceed and defizzed Coke. They drink from paper cups handed to them by volunteers or from plastic squeeze bottles with straws so they don't have to stop to drink.

At a nutritional seminar at Ohio State University in Columbus before the 1992 Olympic trials, Edward F. Coyle, Ph.D., of the Department of Kinesiology at the University of Texas at Austin, suggested that for efficient thermal regulation on a hot day a runner may need to drink 1000 milliliters of fluid an hour. That's a full liter! *Nearly one quart!* If you're a three- or four-hour marathoner, that would mean drinking three or four quart bottles while running at top speed. I've done it under controlled conditions in an exercise laboratory, running on a treadmill with someone handing me a plastic bottle with a straw every five minutes, and it's not easy. It took all my willpower to keep drinking as my belly filled with fluids and my mind sent signals that I no longer was thirsty. Yet that's what Dr. Coyle claims you need to do if you expect the best possible performance.

Learning How to Drink

That is why I plotted those water stops. Not only would it make that Sunday's 20-miler more comfortable, but it would teach those in my class how to drink and how often to drink and underscore the importance of proper fluid replacement.

No tennis player would start a match without practicing lobs; no golfer would think the game complete without learning how to pitch from a sand trap. And no runner should enter a marathon without figuring out how and when to drink.

It's definitely not easy. Unless you grasp cups carefully, you can spill half of the contents on the ground. If you gulp too quickly, you can spend the next mile coughing and gasping. If you dawdle at aid stations, you can waste precious seconds. And if you gulp down a replacement drink you aren't used to, it might make you nauseous.

Drinking on the run is a science—and so we practice. Following the lawn sprinkler at mile 12, I began to falter. Since the start, I had been running with John Ryder, a mail carrier who coaches part-time at one of the local high schools. We had been chatting easily about our teams until we began pushing the pace about halfway into the run. (When that happens in a workout, I usually blame the other runner, and he blames me.) But now I found myself falling five to ten yards behind Ryder as we ran along a straight stretch leading out of Beverly Shores. He started to slow his pace slightly to avoid leaving me.

Mark McGrath was ready with a plastic bottle of Gatorade at mile 14. Tilting the bottle, I inhaled its contents with one breath. Then I ran off without waiting for Ryder, hoping I could gain enough yards to keep up with him until the next water stop in another mile. Sometimes, in the closing stages of runs and races, you motivate yourself by simply trying to get from one stop to another.

But within minutes, my strength returned. My stride lengthened. Life seemed brighter. When Ryder caught me, we pushed on at an even faster pace. It felt as though my body had readily absorbed energy from the drink, allowing me a few more miles reprieve.

I held the pace another four miles before faltering. By that time, I was less than two miles from home, an easy jog in.

Twenty miles in a workout is not 26 in a race, but with sufficient rest and my practiced approach to drinking often, I knew I just might survive that next marathon, and the one after that.

Drinking for Survival

Drinking on the run is necessary for survival. When the weather is warm, runners sweat. We sweat even during cool weather, particularly if we are overdressed. If we sweat too much, we dehydrate. If we become dehydrated, body temperature rises and our performance drops. Too high a body temperature can result in heat prostration, or death.

Most people sweat efficiently and adapt quite well to changes in temperature. It is only when we do extreme activities like run marathons that we have to worry about taking in enough liquid to balance losses from sweat. The average sedentary person loses two quarts of water a day under normal temperature conditions, but a marathoner can sweat away that much in half an hour, according to Lawrence E. Armstrong, Ph.D., of the University of Connecticut.

Alberto Salazar, for example, lost *12 pounds* and placed a sub-par 15th in the 1984 Olympic marathon. "Without doubt, running marathons results in tremendous dehydration," states Peter B. Raven, Ph.D., a physiology professor at the Texas School of Osteopathic Medicine.

Nevertheless, sweating is a natural effect of exercise. "Every muscle is a tiny furnace that produces heat," writes Gabe Mirkin, M.D., in *The Sportsmedicine Book*. Muscles convert fuel to energy very inefficiently, resulting in excess heat that must be eliminated to keep the body from overheating.

A part of your brain called the hypothalamus detects the heat rise in the blood as it circulates, raising the body's core temperature. "The brain says sweat, and the body sweats," explains William Fink, a researcher at Ball State University's Human Performance Laboratory in Muncie, Indiana.

Perspiration begins almost immediately when we start to run, emerging through glands so numerous that an area of skin the size of a quarter contains a hundred. (Our bodies have between two and four million sweat glands.) The rise in body temperature triggers the production and excretion of sweat. As sweat evaporates from the skin, you cool off. This is called thermoregulation, and when it works right it's an effective heating and air conditioning system.

Not everybody's system functions effectively, however. In a running class I taught in Dowagiac, Michigan, in the early 1980s, there was a woman named Joyce who essentially did not sweat. Some people might consider that an advantage, but not if you're a runner. Joyce's inability to sweat normally caused her to overheat so quickly that even on a cool day, she couldn't run farther than three miles. For Joyce to run a marathon would have been an impossibility.

Alberto Salazar had another problem. He had tremendous willpower and could push himself past the point where lesser runners would quit. Tested in Dr. David Costill's lab at Ball State University, he kept running on the treadmill at the point of maximum oxygen uptake much longer than any other runner. But that drive got Salazar into trouble. On two occasions at the peak of his career—once at the Falmouth Road Race and another time at the Boston Marathon—he collapsed after winning fast races and had to receive fluids intravenously.

The Science of Sweat

As Salazar discovered, what scientists refer to as effective thermoregulation occurs at the expense of body fluids. The hotter it is, the more you sweat. "If sweat loss is not replaced during exercise," says Robert Murray, Ph.D., a consultant for the Quaker Oats Company, "the resulting dehydration compromises cardiovascular and thermoregulatory function, increases the risk of heat illness and impairs exercise performance."

Dehydration reduces central blood volume. This prompts the body to decrease both blood flow and sweating in an attempt to conserve body fluids. Under these circumstances, heat loss drops and the body temperature can rise to dangerous levels unless you stop running—and maybe even then, if you fail to get out of the sun.

You can't adapt to dehydration, explains Dr. Murray, but living and training in hot environments can help you *avoid* dehydration. Your blood volume expands and your sweat glands conserve sodium, says Dr. Murray. "This helps assure that cardiovascular and thermoregulatory function can be maintained during exercise in the heat," he says.

What Dr. Murray is saying is that we can train ourselves to utilize fluids more efficiently. Humans are *homeotherms* who need to maintain a constant temperature; we're warm-blooded rather than cold-blooded. An internal temperature of 98.6°F is considered normal. Your body temperature drops *below* normal (called hypothermia) if you stay out too long in the cold or wear insufficient clothes. Your temperature rises *above* normal (hyperthermia) when you start to exercise. It also rises if you get the flu or a similar infection, one reason why it's not a good idea to exercise to excess—or even at all—when you're ill.

Hypothermia normally is not a problem for marathoners—except occasionally on cold days when the runner feels less urge to drink and/or slows drastically in the last miles. (Drinking helps keep you warm as well as keep you cool.)

Hyperthermia is more of a problem. There are two types of sweat glands: apocrine and eccrine. Apocrine glands don't concern marathoners. Those are the "nervous" or "sexual" glands, located mostly in the armpits and around the genital organs. Scientists don't entirely understand their function but suspect they serve some purpose related to sexual attraction.

The eccrine gland, however, keeps us cool. Even though we begin sweating almost immediately as a response to exercise, it may be ten minutes or more before our skin becomes moist enough to notice. On hot but dry days, you may not realize you are sweating, because the moisture evaporates quickly.

Normally, sweat is very dilute water, containing only about one-tenth of a percent electrolytes: mostly sodium chloride and some potassium. There has been some suggestion that perspiration is one of the body's means of ridding the bloodstream of waste products, including lactic acid. Not true. The prime function of the eccrine glands is keeping us cool.

Cooling occurs when sweat evaporates from the body surface. "Evaporation is important," explains Dr. Raven. "The blood flows to the surface and transfers its heat by conduction."

During exercise, the body usually produces more heat than you can get rid of by sweating. A marathoner's body temperature gradually rises 3° or 4° to 102°, an efficient level for energy utilization. At this point, our air conditioning system is in sync with the environment and we perform well. If the weather is too hot or too humid, or we become dehydrated—resulting in a drop in sweat production—the body's temperature soars to dangerous levels. Muscles do not perform efficiently at temperatures too high (104° and up), so that slows us down. This is an important defense mechanism, because if we fail to sweat and our core temperature rises past 108°, we may suffer heatstroke, a potentially serious problem that can cause headaches and dizziness, and in extreme cases convulsions, unconsciousness and death.

The body's ability to safely regulate its internal temperature while exercising is influenced by four factors: the environment, exercise intensity, clothing and the athlete's level of fitness and acclimatization. You can train yourself to resist both cold and hot weather, but extremes of either can cause problems.

Effective Sweating

Let's eliminate one myth. Although Joyce in my running class virtually did not sweat, in general women sweat as much as men. The suspicion that women's air conditioning systems function less efficiently than men's was one excuse the International Olympic Committee offered for resisting the addition of the marathon or any other long-distance race for women to the Olympic Games.

One person who helped disprove this myth has a particularly appropriate name: Barbara L. Drinkwater, Ph.D., of the Department of Medicine at Pacific Medical Center in Seattle, Washington. In 1977, Dr. Drinkwater asked a number of female runners, including one world record holder, to exercise for two hours in an environmental chamber at 118°. "They came out looking like they had climbed out of a swimming pool," Dr. Drinkwater recalls.

Yes, women sweat and, in fact, have more sweat glands than men. In some studies involving men and women, men did sweat more, but Dr. Drinkwater suspects that's because the men and women compared didn't all have comparable weights and oxygen uptake levels.

Regardless of your sex, conditioning improves your ability to sweat. Carl Gisolfi, Ph.D., an exercise physiologist at the University of Iowa, believes that we can increase our heat tolerance 50 percent by conditioning. According to Dr. Gisolfi, you train your sweat glands to function more efficiently by using them.

Acclimatization also improves our ability to tolerate heat. That is why marathoners experience more problems when the weather turns hot at Boston in the spring than at New York in the fall. By New York, they've had an entire summer to become acclimatized.

One year at the Shamrock Shuffle, a popular 8-K race held in Chicago each March, a freak warm spell raised the temperature to an unseasonal 70°. I was astounded to see runners starting the race in tights and jackets, even cotton sweat suits—clothing they had worn through the winter. Most finished the race sweaty and bedraggled, with jackets wrapped around their waists. Several overheated runners were taken to the hospital. A midsummer race with 70° temperatures, however, would have caused few problems. Runners would have been conditioned both physically and psychologically to tolerate the heat.

Buddy Edelen sometimes wore three sweat suits while training for the 1964 Olympic marathon trials to simulate hot conditions. Sure enough, temperatures rose into the 90s during the May trials in Yonkers, New York, and Edelen soundly beat his rivals. Later Olympic marathoners Ron Daws of Minnesota and Benji Durden of Colorado adopted Edelen's training strategy with success.

Tips to Stay Cool

Other than training in multiple sweat suits, what strategies can runners use to prevent heat problems? Let's talk first about practice. Here are some training tips for proper hydration.

Drink before running. Drink adequately and drink often. Dr. Murray recommends drinking 16 ounces of water an hour before training: "Excess body water will be passed as urine before practice begins," he says. Marathoner Doug Kurtis says that he never passes a water fountain at work without stopping for at least a quick drink.

Drink while you run. For years, an old-fashioned notion among coaches was that drinking was for sissies; today's more knowledgeable coaches realize their athletes practice and play better if allowed time to drink. That was the motivation behind the development of Gatorade, a replacement drink formulated for University of Florida football players. Runners need to drink frequently during practice, especially during warm weather. You'll run faster and recover faster. Most runners quickly become adept at locating available water in their neighborhood. I sometimes carry coins in my shorts if I know I'll be passing a soft drink machine.

I live on Lake Shore Drive in Michigan City, the town's most popular route for joggers, bikers and walkers. When I recently added an extra parking space in front of my house, I asked the landscaper to install a water fountain. My popularity in the neighborhood soared as those exercising stopped to cool off.

Drink after running. Most runners don't need to be told this. Their natural instinct sends them immediately to the water fountain or refrigerator. But even after your initial thirst is quenched, you still may be dehydrated. One way of evaluating your intake is to check the color of your urine. If it's yellow, you probably need to keep drinking. Clear urine is a sign of good hydration. Another clue is body weight. If your weight is abnormally low following a long run on a hot day, don't congratulate yourself that you are losing weight; you're most likely badly dehydrated.

Run when it's cool. Because of my flexible schedule as a writer, I can choose my running times. During the winter, I usually train at midday, because it's warmer. During the summer, I switch to running at dawn, before it gets too hot. Running in the evening is slightly less satisfactory because it can still be hot and humid. And running in the dark has its own perils. You may need to do some hot-weather running to acclimatize yourself for races, but you don't want extreme temperatures to affect the quality of your training. I've run at 4:00 in the afternoon near my brother-in-law's house in Mesa, Arizona, when the temperature was 104°. I didn't run far, and I didn't run fast, but I ran— partly to prove I could do it. But I was glad I didn't have to run in those conditions every day.

Shift your training. The message in my earlier book, *Run Fast,* was, "If you want to run fast, you have to run fast." Every coach will tell you that one secret to success—even in the marathon—is speedwork. The best time for speedwork is the summer, when the warm weather helps warm your muscles so you're less likely to suffer injuries. You can train on the track, never more than a short sprint from the water fountain. Short, intense workouts can get you just as hot as long, slow ones, but you'll be closer to home if you do overheat.

Beware of the sun. Wear a hat. Every runner should own a sloppy, floppy, cotton-billed hat that can be used to douse yourself with water when you stop at water fountains. I have one plus another hat with a built-in sweatband, useful for keeping sweat out of your eyes. Particularly in spring, you may want to use sunscreen to protect vulnerable areas, such as your face, shoulders and the front of your legs. Apply the sunscreen half an hour before you run to let it be absorbed, then apply more. Wash your hands thoroughly to avoid rubbing the lotion into your eyes if you wipe your forehead—it can sting badly.

Don't overestimate your ability. Realize that you can't run as fast when it's warm. Don't expect to achieve a preplanned time, and don't be afraid to bail out early when you're starting to overheat.

I learned that lesson the hard way. During the prime of my running career, I set out one morning determined to run at a 5:30 pace on a long run without realizing temperatures were climbing through the 80s. I finished the workout, but barely jogging. Two days later, I came down with a knee injury, which I attributed to my still-dehydrated state: I'm convinced my body lacked sufficient fluid to lubricate the joints. Whether or not that theory is true, it's certain that you can't ignore Mother Nature while running in the heat. Warm-weather training must of necessity be a compromise. But if you learn to live with the heat, you can survive and condition yourself for any type of weather.

Drinking during the Race

Drinking during a marathon race is almost a separate subject, because in addition to your need to stay cool, you also need to adopt a strategy that permits you to refuel on the run. You need energy as well as fluid replacement.

Timing your prerace hydration also can be tricky. I recommend that runners drink as frequently as possible until two hours before the race—then stop until just before the race.

Otherwise they may need to urinate at midrace, an obvious inconvenience. In the last five minutes before the gun, I start drinking again, often downing a 12-ounce soft drink while standing on the starting line, knowing it will be absorbed by the body

Marathon Meals

Unlike cyclists and skiers, most fast marathoners avoid solid foods when they run for a simple reason: It's difficult to eat while moving faster than a 7:00 mile pace.

But Minnesotan Bill Wenmark, who has coached 1,000 runners to finish their first marathon, recommends mid-marathon snacks for people who take longer than three hours to finish. "If you're on the road four or five hours, you're running the equivalent of an ultramarathon," says Wenmark. "You need more energy than you can get from the drinks race directors provide. Someone running an 8:00 pace or slower can take time to eat. Digestion is less a problem than for elite runners." Wenmark recommends saltine crackers and high-energy bars for his back-of-the-packers and positions support crews along the course to provide this extra boost.

What do the scientists say? At Ohio State University, W. Michael Sherman, Ph.D., tested ten cyclists who rode at 70 percent of maximum for 90 minutes, then did the equivalent of a 20-mile time trial. (Their total time approached 2½ hours.) In one trial they ate a specific amount of carbohydrate and in the other they got the carbo in liquid form. "We found no performance difference in their response," reports Dr. Sherman. He adds that in warm weather, liquids certainly would be preferable to solids, because the fluid would help combat dehydration.

Of course, Dr. Sherman admits that his study failed to explore the outer realm of endurance beyond four and five hours where ultramarathoners (and slow marathoners) tread. Conventional wisdom among this breed suggests that food may be as important as drink—if only for the psychological before it reaches the kidneys. That works for me, but every runner has to experiment and come up with their own drinking routine before practice and before races.

"Know what types of replacement beverages will be available

reason that you want something solid in your stomach. First-time marathoners in particular may have a stronger desire to eat solid food than experienced marathoners, who have adapted to a liquids-only diet while racing. Liquids high in sugar also can cause stomach distress—nausea and diarrhea—if you are not used to them.

Solid food for energy replacement was more common in Europe a quarter century ago. When I ran the 1963 Kosice Marathon in Czechoslovakia (an invitational race with only a few finishers slower than three hours), I was surprised to encounter fruits and vegetable soup at the refreshment tables. This was in an era when you were lucky to get water in a U.S. marathon. But at mass European races today, organizers follow the American lead and offer mostly liquids. (It simplifies matters organizationally.)

Inevitably, each runner must determine his or her own regimen. I stick with liquids in running races but have eaten solid food in other endurance events. In triathlons lasting six hours, I've experimented successfully with fruit and candy bars. In a 60-K cross-country ski race, several chocolate chip cookies provided a boost near the end. But during a snowshoe marathon, a combination of soft drinks and candy bars so nauseated me that I failed to finish.

One major logistic problem serves to thwart someone who wants or needs to eat during a marathon. Few marathons provide anything other than liquids. If you're unwilling to carry what you eat in a fanny pack, you may need to enlist a support crew. Most important: If you plan to eat on the run, experiment frequently in practice before you race.

during your race," advises Clark Campbell, a coach and professional triathlete from Lawrence, Kansas. "Then practice with that drink by using it during quality workouts and long distance runs."

You should begin drinking early in the race. If you wait until you get thirsty, you may already have passed several aid stations that could have helped you avoid dehydration. Remember Dr. Coyle's recommendation to drink a quart an hour. Keep that as your goal.

Choosing Your Beverage

Early research in fluid replacement suggested that drinks high in sugar content emptied from the stomach more slowly than water. Then scientists fine-tuned their experiments and determined that fluids with a 6 percent sugar solution emptied from the stomach almost as fast as water. Most replacement drinks offered in major marathons now are formulated at that level. So except for the hottest days, you're better off reaching for the replacement drink at refreshment stations rather than water (unless the sugar in the drink makes you nauseous). Edward F. Coyle, Ph.D., of the University of Texas at Austin, estimates that ingesting 30 to 60 grams of carbohydrates each hour of exercise will generally maintain blood glucose oxidation late in exercise and delay fatigue.

You can reach this level by drinking between 625 and 1250 milliliters (about ⅔ quart to 1¼ quarts) per hour of a beverage that contains between 4 and 8 percent carbohydrates. This could be Coke or various replacement drinks. For races beyond the marathon distance, where energy replacement becomes as important as thermoregulation, supersaturated sugar solutions higher than 8 percent may be necessary. (You can adjust the percentage by varying how much water you mix with powdered replacement drinks—check the directions.)

Dr. Coyle says the largest factor affecting gastric emptying is volume. In other words, the more fluids you can force into your stomach, the faster fluids will empty from the stomach to be absorbed by the body. Dr. Coyle suggests that you may need to take in between 1300 and 1700 milliliters to force 1000 milliliters to be emptied from the stomach during a marathon.

There are certain trade-offs to consider when deciding how much of what liquid to drink. One question is: Are the physical benefits of drinking large volumes of fluid worth the discomfort of making yourself drink so often?

On the hottest days, *yes.*

But the important goal is staying cool. "Any dehydration causes problems," says Dr. Coyle. "None can be tolerated." This is true not only for safety but also for performance. For every liter of fluid lost, your heartbeat will increase eight beats and your core temperature will increase accordingly. As a result, you'll be unable to maintain your race pace. If your goal is safety and performance, there's no question that the closer you match your rate of dehydration, the better.

In the closing stages of the race, water splashed on the body may help you more than water taken into the body. This is because it normally takes 30 minutes for water to migrate through the system to be released as sweat to provide an air conditioning effect. One way to shortcut that system is to pour water directly on your body, permitting it to evaporate. In the last few miles of the race, you're drinking for recovery after the race as much as for performance during it. My motto for the last half hour of running is "water on" as much as "water in."

If you're wearing a hat, pour water onto the hat, allowing it to drip onto your face. Rather than splashing yourself in front, pour water down your back, since it's less likely to flow downward into your shoes and cause blisters. If you pass someone standing beside the road with a water spray, stop to stand under the spray for at least a few seconds rather than running through or around the spray.

The more attention you give to staying cool, the better you'll run. Once you get across the finish line, you'll want to begin drinking immediately to speed your recovery, but that's the subject for another chapter.

CHAPTER 15

Marathon
MIND GAMES

I t was chilly for the Twin Cities Marathon in 1991: a day for tights, long-sleeved tops, earbands and gloves. I brought two gloves with me but lost one on the way to the starting line. To keep both hands warm as I ran, I switched the glove from hand to hand every third mile. It became a game for me, something to think about, something to help chart my progress. I could look forward to the switch each third mile.

In those terms, a marathon is merely eight glove-changes long.

Psychologists have long insisted that the mind is as important as the body when it comes to success in sports, particularly in an event like the marathon where the mind must push the body to extremes. During the glory days of Iron Curtain athletes, sports psychologists were as important as other coaches or trainers in preparing East German and Soviet athletes for competition. The U.S. Olympic Committee now employs psychologists as consultants, as do many professional football and baseball teams. But anyone can use mind games to help get through long-distance events.

I use mind games for survival in the marathon, physically as well as mentally. I divide marathons into fourths and thirds. At 6 miles, I think: "A fourth of the race done." And at 8 miles, "A third." At 10, I console myself: "Double digits." At 16: "Only single digits remain." At 20: "I've passed the Wall." By that time, you're close enough to count down like the liftoff of a rocket: "Six-five-four-three-two-one. I'm done."

But marathon mind games are more than strategies for coping with pain and boredom. According to Charles A. Garfield, author of *Peak Performance,* 60 to 90 percent of success in sports is due to mental factors and psychological mastery. Psychologist Thomas Tutko quotes retired baseball player Maury Wills as saying that success is *all* mental. "There is nothing mystical about the emotional side of sports," claims Dr. Tutko.

Unfortunately, your mind can also work *against* you. One of the coaches responding to my questionnaire commented about a top-ranked woman runner he used to coach: "It's her thinking that keeps her from winning."

Positive Thinking Pays Off

Confidence is an important factor in the mind games athletes play: The power of positive thinking relates to more than success in business. One study of skiers training for the Olympic team showed that those who didn't make the team had negative or tentative feelings about their abilities, while successful candidates were more positive. Does confidence breed success, or were the less successful skiers simply being realistic about their talents? A little bit of both, probably, but consider the cocky attitude of Alpine skier Bill Johnson before he won the 1984 Olympic downhill in Sarajevo: Did Johnson know he had a lock on the gold medal, or was he simply trying to psych himself up?

If the latter, he succeeded, as did British decathlete Daley Thompson, who also boasted of success before the 1984 games. Referring to his chief competitor, Thompson said, "The only way [Jurgen] Hingsen is going to get a gold medal here is to do another event—or steal mine." Thompson prevailed, but Jamaica's Bert Cameron—who had claimed before the games that the 400-meter gold medal already had his name engraved on it—pulled a muscle in a semifinal heat and saw the medal go to another. There's a subtle line between confidence and overconfidence.

When we are confident, we can rationalize away any potential problems; without confidence, even slight threats become magnified.

Confident athletes can relax more easily than ones who feel threatened, but there are tricks to relaxing and eliminating fear. Robert M. Nideffer, Ph.D., a consultant for the U.S. Olympic Committee, recalled watching a diver about to execute a difficult 3½ somersault in pike position off the ten-meter tower. The coach stood below counting down: "Five, four, three, two, one. Go!" The counting, Dr. Nideffer explained, helped the diver redirect his attention away from his anxiety and fear. He likened it to a hypnotic state. Marathoner Tony Sandoval used a similar five-to-zero countdown when he went to bed each night. "It relaxed me and helped me to fall asleep quickly," explains Sandoval.

Visualizing Success

As a steeplechaser, I had my own presleep technique. I would visualize myself hurdling over barriers. It was better, I thought, than the more traditional counting of sheep, but it served another purpose beyond self-hypnosis. I was perfecting my hurdling technique through a technique known as "imaging."

John Syer and Christopher Connolly, in their book *Sporting Body, Sporting Mind,* refer to this same technique as instant *pre*play. They describe one horsewoman who would lock herself in the washroom—the only place she wouldn't be disturbed—immediately before competition to focus on her event. In *Golf My Way,* Jack Nicklaus describes visualizing each shot before he hits it. He first pictures the ball landing where he wants it, then "sees" the ball going there, and finally visualizes himself "making the kind of swing that will turn the previous images into reality." Jon Lugbill, world champion kayaker, pictures himself paddling down white-water rivers and feels this helps his ability to choose the best path through the waves during competition. Runners who want to improve their form similarly can picture themselves running like Olympic champions Gelindo Bordin or Rosa Mota. Tom Grogon, a coach from Cincinnati, Ohio, suggests that runners mentally review the course before any distance race and think about how they will run it.

Another technique is instant *re*play, which Syer and Connolly describe as: "The reverse of instant preplay, it is a visualized review of an action you have just performed." This enables the athlete to imprint a perfect action more deeply in his or her sensory memory. Members of the U.S. weight-lifting team preparing for the Olympics used these techniques. Each weight-lifter had a video tape of his lifts at various meets and in training. As additional meets were filmed, the athletes added new tapes to their collection. With their library of tapes, the athletes could compare their recent lift styles with previous lifts or those of other top lifters filmed during competition.

The Power of Concentration

One way to succeed in sports is to eliminate outside distractions. When that happens, you can more easily relax. Bryant J. Cratty, author of *Psychological Preparation and Athletic Excellence,* believes that relaxation and concentration can be improved in competition if the athlete erects imaginary walls to block off distractions. He suggests that a basketball player visualize partitions in front of the other players and behind the backboard before attempting to shoot a free-throw. Dr. Cratty recommends that a gymnast imagine not only that the gym is empty but that there is a tent over each apparatus. So too should a long-distance runner focus on a narrow corridor of the road ahead.

Dr. Garfield says concentration is important for weight-lifters: "The trained lifter knows that during the few seconds before a lift, total attention must be focused on the bar, and the degree to which this is done is largely determined by how much he really wants to make the lift." Dr. Garfield found that if the lifter's confidence was lacking, his will not intensely focused, he would not be able to muster the control of muscle power necessary for success. The same is true in running.

"The ability to concentrate," says William P. Morgan, Ed.D., "is the single element that separates the merely good athletes from the great ones. Concentration is the hallmark of the elite runner." He says that elite runners succeed because they are totally in tune with their bodies, monitoring all symptoms from the nerve endings.

In contrast, Dr. Morgan found that middle-of-the-pack

marathoners more often thought of other activities (called dissociating) as a means of coping with pain. In addition to possibly
slowing them, Dr. Morgan considers this tactic dangerous: The
runners could ignore important body signals and mindlessly run
themselves into a heatstroke or stress fracture.

Owen Anderson, Ph.D., the editor of *Running Research News,*
defines dissociation as *"ignoring* the sensory feedback you get
from your body while focusing your mind on something outside
yourself." He claims that while dissociation blocks negative messages, prevents boredom and diverts the mind from the pain and
fatigue in the muscles during strenuous running, it can create
some problems if it causes you to fail to take in enough fluid,
relax or exert efficient muscle control. "It's hard to sustain a
coordinated, quality pace unless you concentrate," says Dr.
Anderson.

When I ran marathons near the front of the pack, I always
considered concentration as important an ability as a high VO_2
max. I focused on every stride and was acutely aware of any signals from my body. I always liked the idea of running on scenic
courses—except I almost never saw the scenery. Usually the better I ran, the less I recalled of the surroundings. I'd run the
Boston Marathon a dozen times or more and knew that the
course passed somewhere near Fenway Park, where the Boston
Red Sox played. But I was unaware how near until one year I
covered the race for *Runner's World* and realized that Fenway
Park was right on the course. To have missed it while racing, my
field of vision must have been very narrow.

What Top Runners Do

Other runners agree on the value of concentration. Olympic
marathoner Don Kardong states: "It's absolutely essential that
you concentrate on your competition, monitor your body feedback
and not lose touch with what's happening around you. If you lose
concentration in a good competitive 10-K field, you immediately
drop off the pace. There's never time to think those favorite
thoughts you have on easy training runs."

Greg Meyer, who struggled to regain his form after winning
Boston in 1983, ran several meets in Europe one summer. "I'd

lose concentration for a lap or two," Meyer told me, "and that would get me out of the race. I'd drift off, get gapped and never make it up."

Meyer felt that a series of injuries contributed to his inability to concentrate. "You start focusing on the injuries instead of racing," he said. But it's possible that in winning Boston he had satisfied many of the inner demons that had driven him to success. He may have lost some of his will to win and with it an ability to concentrate.

Dick Buerkle was top ranked in the 5000 in 1974 and set an indoor mile record in 1978. Buerkle noticed that in both years his ability to concentrate was at its highest. "I'd go for an 18-miler every weekend and be totally focused," he recalls. "Other years, I'd find myself daydreaming."

Kardong notes that some distance runners have difficulty switching from roads to track or cross country. He suspects that the biggest factor isn't training, but concentration: "When in an unfamiliar setting, you're distracted by it initially. Later, you adapt."

Bill Rodgers believed concentration must begin before a race. Rodgers avoided warming up with others, preferring to think of the upcoming race. He also believes that the clinics, dinners and social events he attends as part of sponsor commitments diminish his concentration.

During a marathon race Rodgers would think of specific things to help him concentrate: splits, competition, the course, the wind. "If I have a chance to win," he thinks: "What's my best way to race certain individuals?"

Greg Meyer learned he could concentrate better if he ran fartlek rather than straight distance: "Rather than doing mindless 20-milers, you vary the pace, which forces you to pay attention." Sue King, while training for the New York City Marathon, found she could concentrate more by running long runs alone, so the conversation of friends didn't distract her.

Developing Powers of Concentration

So how can you learn to concentrate? How do you focus your mind on the business at foot?

At least one study shows that the average runner can learn to think like the elite. Hein Helgo Schomer of the University of Cape Town in South Africa improved the concentration of a group of non-elite runners. Schomer coached ten non-elite runners for five weeks on how to concentrate. Before coaching, the runners used association (being tuned into their bodies) only 45 percent of the time. By the fifth week, they were associating 70 percent of the time while running, and their average training intensity also rose.

Dr. Anderson states that the average runner probably associates about 30 to 40 percent of the time while running. He considers 60 to 70 percent optimal and 90 to 100 percent necessary for supreme efforts. "Association is clearly a strategy you can use to reach your true potential as a runner," Dr. Anderson says. "Associative thinking can increase your ability to handle strenuous workouts and cope with tough races. While it boosts your aerobic fitness, association probably also minimizes your risk of overtraining by keeping you in tune with how your body is responding to your overall training intensity and volume."

But learning to concentrate takes time. Each spring, once the snow melts, I head for the track for weekly interval sessions to try to regain speed lost after a winter of slow running. When I begin running interval quarters, I know that to run my fastest, I have to concentrate. Yet invariably I'll get on the backstretch and my mind will wander and cause my pace to lag. Only after five or six weeks does my concentration improve to where I can keep my attention on running for a full quarter. My track times then start to drop, convincing me that the improvement results from both stronger muscles and stronger mind.

To hone his ability to concentrate, Dick Buerkle would do long repeats, rather than short ones, running repeat miles between 4:14 and 4:20. "It requires more effort to concentrate for four minutes than for the 27 seconds it takes to run a 200," he says.

Along with Buerkle, I've also found various forms of speedwork—intervals on the track, fartlek in the woods, strides on the grass—the most effective way of improving my concentration. Sometimes I'll head to the golf course several times a week to run a half dozen or more short sprints—not flat-out, but close to the speed I reach in a track mile. I do these "strides" to loosen

The Final Six Miles

Many of the more than 50 coaches who responded to our questionnaire offered various mental strategies for the final six miles, when the marathon gets toughest and where concentration often determines the difference between a good and a bad race.

Frank X. Mari of Toms River, New Jersey, suggested that runners focus on positive thoughts. "Try to catch the next runner in front of you. Remember your hard training and that you are the greatest. Smile."

Tim Nicholls of Pembroke Pines, Florida, says: "Stick with someone in the race. Ask yourself how badly you want it."

Tom Grogon of Cincinnati advises: "Toward the end, concentrate on passing as many runners as possible. As soon as you pass one competitor, concentrate on reeling in the next. Think of the world as ending right after the race, thus there is no reason not to put everything into it."

David Cowein of Morrilton, Arkansas, says: "In the last six miles, think of how many times you've run a 10-K before. Focus on your achievements. You've trained hard. You deserve your best. You're nearly through. Tell yourself how tough you are."

As you run more marathons, you'll determine what mental strategies work best to get you through those final six miles.

my muscles for other, longer and tougher workouts. Invariably I return from the golf course running much faster, my mind totally focused.

I have difficulty concentrating during track workouts, and particularly on distance runs, but I usually manage to get my act together for important races: Competition tends to focus my mind. Maybe that's why I achieve speeds in competition that are beyond my reach in training.

Blocking Out Mind Drift

How do you get mind and body in tune to run long distances faster? Here are several tips to help you block out mind drift.

Prepare yourself to run. Have a game plan for workouts and particularly for important races. Where are you going to run? How fast? How far? Against whom? Get yourself in a running frame of mind. Learn to relax. A regular warm-up routine before running can get you into the mood to perform. Find a routine that works best for you—whether chanting a mantra or stretching—and stick with it.

Discover how your body works. While running fast, try to be aware of what the various parts of your body are doing. Can you discover what it feels like to run smoothly? If so, you may be able to duplicate that feeling on other occasions. Remember: Given equal athletic skills, the ability to concentrate separates the merely good runners from the great ones.

Practice instant preplay and replay. If you can imagine before running how top runners run successfully—preplay—you're halfway to emulating them. Practice running mentally as well as physically. Replay as well. When you run well, remember how you ran. Fix that image in your memory, adding it to your mental video library.

Head for the track. Running against the clock and attempting to match preset goals forces you to concentrate. Learning to adjust to the track's rhythm—running turns, for example—also helps, as do fartlek and other forms of speedwork done elsewhere.

Plan days of maximum concentration. Every workout need not be fully focused, but select one or more days each week to practice concentration. Racing, particularly track or cross-country races, also may help focus your mind.

Avoid race-day distractions. Friends, traffic or dogs can all distract you from the act and art of running. Run solo when you can to improve your concentration. If you want to succeed with your race plan, keep conversation to a minimum even if you're running with a friend.

Talk to yourself. Cardiologist Paul Thompson, M.D., believes runners need pep talks. "I talk to myself when I train," he says.

"The year I ran best at Boston, I focused on what to tell myself during those last few miles when it hurts." Thompson placed 16th at Boston in 1976 by telling himself, "Keep going," and "I'm a tough dude."

Focus hardest when it counts most. If you find it difficult to concentrate the full 26 miles of a marathon, save your focus for the miles when you need it the most. Don Kardong used to dissociate the first half of the race, then associate the second half. "My mind wanders at times," admits Doug Kurtis. "I like to look around and check the scenery, but I particularly try to focus late in the race, especially when I know a sub-2:20 is on the line."

Concentration can't compensate for lack of training or basic ability, but it can help you maximize your potential.

CHAPTER 16

MILE 27

The most important mile of the marathon may be mile number 27, the one you walk to the hotel. Shortly after finishing the Boston Marathon a few years ago, I sat huddled on a bench in Copley Square, wrapped in an aluminum blanket, with a soft drink in one hand and in the other a cup of frozen yogurt that I was too nauseated to eat. I cursed having stayed at a hotel whose distance from the finish line would require another mile's walk—a 27th mile, so to speak—before I could end that day's marathon experience.

Yet 15 minutes later, halfway to the hotel, frozen yogurt consumed, sipping a second soft drink, I felt my energy returning. I knew I would recover and eventually run 26 miles again.

That 27th mile is particularly important when it comes to speeding postmarathon recovery, so that you can run and race again. Your actions during the first five seconds after crossing the line may be crucial to your recovery—as are the next five minutes, the next five hours, the next five days and even the next five weeks. Postmarathon recovery is something many runners pay scant attention to. But by organizing your postrace plans as well as you organize your prerace plans, you can recover faster and more comfortably and minimize future injuries.

Minimizing the Damage

"Runners need to take responsibility for the health of their muscles, not just how fast they go," warns Linda Jaros, a massage therapist from Dedham, Massachusetts, whose clients include Bill Rodgers and Joan Benoit Samuelson. "Recovery has to become an integral part of their training."

Indeed, recovery may be the toughest skill for a marathon runner to master. How do you snap back after more than 26 hard miles on the road? Are fatigued and sore muscles inevitable, or are there strategies that will make marathon recovery not only faster but less painful? What secrets can we learn both from elite and ordinary marathoners that will allow a quick return to full training—and the next starting line? What do scientists suggest based on laboratory research, not only for the morning after but for the week after?

David L. Costill, Ph.D., director of the Human Performance Laboratory at Ball State University in Muncie, Indiana, has researched the damage marathons do to the body, both in the lab and on the road. In numerous studies, Dr. Costill has reviewed the postrace drinking, eating and training habits of marathoners. Dr. Costill's suggestions for recovery: Drink plenty of fluids, carbo-load after the race and don't start running again too soon. "A lot of things happen to the body as a result of running the marathon," he says. "You become overheated, dehydrated and muscle-depleted. Your hormonal milieu gets thrown out of whack, and you traumatize your muscles. You have to bide your time to get your body back in balance."

Since 1974, Jack H. Scaff, Jr., M.D., has supervised the Honolulu Marathon Clinic, a group that meets Sundays in Kapiolani Park to train for the marathon. After watching his group's recuperative efforts after the race, Dr. Scaff commented, "The runners felt so good about their achievement, they would bounce back too soon. The rate of injuries was exponential. We finally canceled the clinic for three months following the marathon to try and get the runners to take it easy."

Benji Durden of Boulder, Colorado, who qualified for the boycotted 1980 Olympics, has observed the effects of marathon running on the body as a runner and as a coach of others, including 2:26:40 marathoner Kim Jones. Durden recalls running a 2:15 at Boston in 1978—cutting four minutes off his best time—then spraining an ankle the following week. "My body had not fully recovered," he notes. While conceding that total rest may be the best postmarathon prescription, Durden contends that runners may have conflicting psychological needs. "As a coach I try to accept the best advice from the scientists and adapt it based on a combination of intuition and experience," he says.

Keep Moving

Want to recover as rapidly as possible following your next marathon? First, don't stop as soon as you cross the finish line. You may have no choice, particularly at major races where you will be prodded to jog and walk through the finish chute, after which you run a gauntlet that includes having various items pressed onto you: your medal, fluids and food, an aluminum blanket and your gear brought from the starting line. Having accepted all this, you may need to walk what seems an unconscionably long distance to be greeted by friends and family.

Whether prodded or not, keep moving to allow your stressed system a chance to gradually attain a steady state and also to avoid what Dr. Scaff calls, "the postrace collapse phenomenon." This, he says, is when "a runner looks good coming across the finish line, sits down too soon, then 20 minutes later must be taken to the first aid tent with heatstroke or cramps." Blood pressure also can drop too quickly, sometimes with disastrous results. "Walking around a bit seems to prevent this from happening," says Dr. Scaff.

How much you walk depends on your condition at the end of the race. "If your body is telling you to collapse in a heap, walking around is not easy," says Dr. Costill. "But continuing to move for a while will maintain your circulation, keeping the blood pumping through the muscles. This should aid short-term recovery."

Warning: Don't take the advice to keep moving to excess. Many compulsive runners feel the need to "cool down" by jogging a mile or two, even after a marathon. While this may make sense following a 10-K race, it does not after a 42.2-K race. No scientific studies have shown *any* benefits from postrace running. You simply increase your chance of injury by continuing to run.

Drink Up

As long as you're walking, head in the direction of the tables with fluids. All the experts—scientists and experienced marathoners alike—advise an *immediate* and *continuing* effort to replace the several liters of liquid your system has shed during 26 miles on the road. Grab the first cup of liquid thrust into your hand and start sipping at once, no matter how nauseated you feel.

Dr. Scaff recommends sipping at the rate of ½ ounce a minute. And while going about other recuperative activities for the next several hours, keep a drink in your hand and continue drinking. Like most experts, Dr. Costill emphasizes that human thirst is not an accurate gauge of dehydration. "Drink more than you desire," he advises.

If the first cup thrust into your hand is water, accept it thankfully and sip on it, but look for the table where they have drinks with at least some dilute form of sugar, whether in a so-called replacement drink (such as E.R.G. or Exceed), a soft drink or a fruit drink. While your primary need is to replace fluids, you also have depleted your muscles of glycogen and need to replace that as well. "Try to get your blood sugar back to normal as quickly as possible," says Durden.

The best time for glycogen replacement, according to research by Edward F. Coyle, Ph.D., at the University of Texas at Austin, is the first two hours after the race. "The muscles absorb glycogen like a sponge," says Dr. Coyle. "Four and six hours after the race, the absorption rate starts to decline." Nutritionists may argue that, generally speaking, fruit drinks (because they contain vitamins and minerals) are superior to sugar drinks—and this certainly is true—but Dr. Costill claims that when it comes to glycogen replacement the body doesn't know the difference between one sugar and another.

Top marathoner Doug Kurtis doesn't mind having to undergo drug testing as a prizewinner. In order to provide the necessary urine specimen, Kurtis finds he must drink steadily for two hours. "That forces me to ingest a lot of fluids," says Kurtis. "I feel that helps my recovery."

Two postmarathon drinks to avoid: diet soft drinks, because they provide no glucose boost (having just burned approximately 2,600 calories, your goal should *not* be weight loss) and alcoholic beverages, because they serve as a diuretic. That postrace beer may taste good, but it will have an eventual negative effect on fluid balance. If you drink a beer, do so only after previously ingesting twice the volume of other fluids.

Get Off Your Feet

After spending the first five or ten minutes walking around and obtaining something to drink, get off your feet. Listen to your body, "Do what it tells you to do," says Dr. Costill. "Get horizontal." Pick a comfortable spot, preferably in the shade, and elevate your feet, easing the flow of blood to the heart. Dr. Costill speculates that some of the muscle soreness and stiffness experienced immediately after the race may be related to edema, swelling caused by intermuscular pressure of accumulated fluids in the lower legs. "Elevating the legs may speed recovery," he suggests.

You can assist this recovery with gentle self-massage. But don't knead; instead, stroke your leg muscles gently toward the heart. Durden and New York City marathon winner Priscilla Welch recommend massaging with ice to reduce the edema. Hosing your legs with cold water is another method.

Bill Rodgers, four-time winner of both the Boston and New York City marathons, likes to do some postrace stretching while lying down. If you choose to do the same, don't stretch excessively. Your muscles most likely are stiff and damaged; you don't want to traumatize them further.

Some researchers even question the value of stretching. A study at the University of Texas at Tyler indicated that static stretching failed to prevent muscle soreness later. Researchers Katherine C. Buroker and James A. Schwane, Ph.D., concede that stretching helps maintain flexibility but say that immediately after strenuous exercise is the wrong time for it. When Dr. Scaff surveyed members of his Honolulu Marathon Clinic, he discovered that those who stretched most also suffered the most injuries. Scientists remain divided on the value of stretching, so your best bet is to keep any stretching short and simple after a marathon.

While resting, continue to sip fluids—this is still your primary recovery strategy. Using a bent straw makes it easier to drink while horizontal.

Begin to Refuel

Your immediate concern may have been fluid replacement, but within an hour after the race, you should begin shifting to more solid foods. This may be particularly important if sugar from replacement drinks makes you nauseated, as food can slow down sugar absorption to help prevent the nausea. Ken Young of Tucson, Arizona, a top trail runner and coach of 2:11 marathoner Don Janicki, likes saltine crackers to help settle his stomach. Fruit is a good start, particularly bananas because they are easy to digest and are a good source of lost potassium. (Don't become obsessed with instant mineral replacement, however; eating several well-balanced meals within the next 24 hours will take care of electrolytes lost through sweating.)

"Food has real nutritional value, whereas sports drinks are just sugar," says Nancy Clark, R.D., author of *The Athlete's Kitchen* and *Nancy Clark's Sports Nutrition Guidebook* and nutritionist with SportsMedicine Brookline in Boston, Massachusetts. Clark recommends fruit or yogurt (frozen and otherwise) as a superior snack to cookies or candy bars. Research by Dr. Coyle indicates that one gram of carbohydrate per kilogram of body weight per hour is necessary for most efficient glycogen replacement. That translates to 2 calories per pound, or 300 calories for a 150-pound runner. Clark suggests that a marathoner drink a glass of orange juice and eat one banana and a cup of yogurt the first hour, then repeat that the second hour.

As a practical matter, I'll grab anything handy, particularly those chocolate-chip cookies at the end of the table. Immediately after a marathon, I'm like a shark feeding. Anything in close range of my mouth gets consumed.

Consider Massage

Many major marathons provide massage tents with teams of trained massage therapists ready to provide a soothing rubdown. According to Linda Jaros, massage helps push waste products from the muscles into the blood system for recirculation. Most runners find they feel better after a full-body massage.

Jaros cautions against a too-early or too-strenuous massage after a marathon, however. Early finishers sometimes head straight to the massage tent to beat the crowd, but it's preferable to wait 45 minutes, giving yourself time to rehydrate and cool down. And don't allow therapists to poke and probe your muscles as vigorously as they might during a regular session. The best postmarathon massage, according to therapist Rich Phaigh of Eugene, Oregon, begins with the lower back and buttocks to relax those muscles and get intramuscular fluids flowing, then works gently on the legs with long, flowing motions toward the heart. If the massage hurts, ask the therapist to be more gentle; if it still hurts, thank the therapist graciously and get off the table.

For those with a regular massage therapist, the best time for a massage may be 24 to 48 hours after the race, a time when muscle soreness usually peaks. In preparing for the Sunburst Marathon, I scheduled appointments with my regular massage therapist the afternoon before the race *and* two days after.

Avoid hot baths or showers that may increase inflammation and unnecessarily elevate your body temperature. That bubbling whirlpool back at the motel may look inviting, but leave it to the kids. Opt for a *cool* shower. "Getting your body temperature back down will help you recover faster," says Dr. Costill. Jaros suggests a cold bath followed by a warm (not hot) shower. Aspirin should be avoided, according to Tufts University research. While it may reduce the pain of sore muscles, it also prolongs the time of damage repair.

Recovery Continues at Home

Most marathoners don't want to abandon the scene of battle too rapidly. Admittedly, part of the enjoyment of marathoning is hanging around to see old friends and rivals, cheering their finishes and swapping stories about the miles just covered. Don't deny yourself the opportunity to wallow a while in the joy of your accomplishment.

But after you've gotten home and showered, jump into bed. Even if you have difficulty sleeping, at least rest for one or two hours. Then get up: It's time for more food.

Three or four hours after finishing, sit down to a full meal. Dr. Costill claims that carbohydrates should still be the food of choice. "Nutritionally, your first meal after the marathon should resemble your last meal before," he says. Sound advice, although many marathoners rebel against having to look at one more plate of pasta and instead indulge a sudden craving for protein. "I'm not afraid to eat a hamburger after a marathon," confesses Doug Kurtis. "It almost feels like a reward." Bill Rodgers recalls going to a restaurant one year after placing third in the Boston Marathon and eating a hamburger followed by a hot fudge sundae. He also fondly recalls family victory celebrations at his store with picnic lunches of chicken sandwiches supplied by his mother.

But remember that spaghetti isn't the only form of carbohydrate. "Even high-carbohydrate diets have some protein," says Clark. "Your body needs to rebuild protein, so have your chicken or steak or fish, but start with some minestrone soup. Add some extra potatoes, rolls and juice. The secret in anything you eat is moderation. Don't focus on the meat; focus on the carbohydrates that can accompany the meat."

Take a Break

Once home, too many marathoners make the mistake of resuming training too soon. They may fear getting out of shape or feel that some easy jogging will help speed their recovery. Kurtis always runs the next day, "even if only to limp through a mile"—but most of us don't have his capabilities. The body of someone used to 105-mile training weeks and as many as a dozen marathons a year functions differently than that of an ordinary runner.

Research by Dr. Costill suggests that recovery is speeded and conditioning is not affected if you do nothing for seven to ten days after the race. Repeat: For the week after your marathon, *do nothing!*

Durden, however, thinks it's all right to resume *easy* running by the fourth day. He wouldn't recommend the cross-training used by some recuperating marathoners. "When I say rest, I mean rest," he says. "Not Nautilus. Not exercycling. Not swimming. Not walking. You rest! I've worked with a few athletes who thought rest meant everything except run."

Moving in the pool is another matter. It may comfort the muscles if you immerse yourself in water and use gentle, nonaerobic movements to stretch and relax your arms and legs. But don't start paddling, because you will simply delay recovery by burning more glycogen.

Ease Back into Training

Once back with running, don't run too hard or too fast too soon. Dr. Scaff recommends the 10 percent rule: No more than 10 percent of your total mileage can be spent in racing or speedwork. "After you've run a marathon, you need 260 miles of training before you enter your next event or start doing speedwork," says Dr. Scaff. "For someone running 30 to 40 miles a week, that means six to eight weeks of recovery running. Someone used to higher mileage probably recovers sooner."

Bill Rodgers took his time coming back after marathons. "Slowly, over a period of weeks, I'd build back to regular mileage," says Rodgers. "I'd stick with once-a-day training for a while. No speed or long runs for at least two or three weeks."

Particularly after a good performance, runners need to avoid the urge to come back too soon. It's tempting to increase training under the theory that more work may mean still better times. "You end up pushing yourself too hard," warns Durden. "You may get away with it for four to six weeks, then you collapse, get injured, get sick, or feel stale and overtrained. The period immediately after a good marathon is when you need to be especially cautious about your training."

Russell H. Pate, Ph.D., chairman of the Department of Exercise Science at the University of South Carolina, developed a two-week recovery method through trial and error. "I'd have very minimal activity for two to three days after the race, still modest running for the remainder of the first week, then over the second week gradually build to near my normal training loads. By the third week, I'd be ready to run hard again." But on one occasion when he felt good after three days and resumed heavy training too quickly, three weeks later he had a breakdown featuring minor injuries and fatigue. "I learned the hard way to put the brakes on," Dr. Pate recalls.

"Studies now show you do, indeed, damage the muscle, creating microtrauma in muscle fibers with activities like marathon running," he says. "No one knows what we do to the connective tissue and skeleton, but I suspect there's trauma there also. Since scientists do not yet know precisely how much time is needed for such trauma to be reversed, it's smart for runners to give themselves plenty of time with minimal running to let that healing process occur."

None of the experts—neither scientists, coaches nor experienced road runners—can offer an exact formula for marathon recovery. Too many factors are involved, from the condition of the athlete going into the race to the conditions of the race itself. Hilly courses, particularly those with downhills near the end such as Boston, do more muscle damage than flat courses. Extremes of heat or cold slow the recovery process. And runners who go out too fast and crash usually have more difficulty recovering than those who run an even pace.

"Nature takes care of us," says Dr. Costill. "Time heals most of the damage done in the marathon." Through careful attention to the 27th mile, most of us will be back on the road again, looking forward to our next trip to the starting line.

CHAPTER 17

Top Coaches'
TRAINING
PLANS

Many coaches resist providing formula training plans. Those coaches reason—correctly—that each runner is different. Not only do runners differ in their ability (some can run a marathon in just over two hours; others take more than five or six hours), but those runners have different *types* of ability. Because of variations in genetic makeup, some people respond better to speedwork, some better to long distance.

"I hate the cookbook recipe approach implied in published training schedules," says marathon coach Bill Wenmark, and that sentiment is shared by many.

The best approach for runners is to have a knowledgeable coach such as Wenmark or the other coaches who contributed information to this book. That coach can individualize a training schedule and—perhaps most important—modify that training schedule on a week-by-week and day-by-day basis. The ideal situation certainly is to have a good coach looking over your shoulder as you run.

Nevertheless, runners can learn by examining the training schedules of other runners and by analyzing the kinds of training plans coaches prescribe for beginning, experienced and elite marathoners. With that in mind, I asked seven top coaches to provide training plans for runners at each of those three levels. Their plans, which appear on the following pages, are worth reviewing, with special note of both differences and similarities. (All these plans would require that beginning marathoners have enough of a training base to be able to comfortably run the distances listed.)

Lee Fidler
Stone Mountain, Georgia

Lee Fidler is a running consultant. As a competitive runner, he has personal bests of 30:03 for 10,000 meters and 2:15:04 for the marathon. Fidler finished five times in the top 20 at Boston and competed in three Olympic marathon trials. Marathoners he has coached include Steve Oliver (2:20:37), Lyle Parker (2:20:43), Lucia Geraci (2:45:55), Sue Parker (2:50:06) and Kim Nelson (2:57:35).

Fidler's training plans:

Novice Marathoners
Sunday: Long run—1:30 to 1:45
Monday: Rest
Tuesday: 30 minutes
Wednesday: 4 × 800; 2:00 rest between
Thursday: 30 minutes
Friday: 30 minutes
Saturday: Rest

Experienced Marathoners
Sunday: Long run—1:30 to 1:45
Monday: 30 minutes
Tuesday: 0 to 45 minutes
Wednesday (A.M.): 4 miles; **(P.M.):** 6 × 800; 1:30 rest between
Thursday: 30 to 40 minutes
Friday: 60 to 80 minutes
Saturday: 30 to 40 minutes

Elite Marathoners
Sunday: Long run—2 to 3 hours
Monday: 45 to 60 minutes, easy
Tuesday (A.M.): 60 to 70 minutes; **(P.M.):** 30 to 45 minutes

Wednesday: 45 to 60 minutes, easy
Thursday (A.M.): 3-mile warm-up; 6 × 800; 1:30 rest between; 4-mile cool-down; **(P.M.):** 6 miles, easy
Friday: 45 to 60 minutes, easy
Saturday: 60 to 70 minutes

Tip: Be alert to body signals. Program rest into your training. Recover from one hard workout before proceeding to the next.

Susan Kinsey
La Mesa, California

Susan Kinsey is a personal trainer and coach. In 1977, Kinsey placed eighth (first American) in the world cross-country championships. She has run the 10,000 in 33:42 and the marathon in 2:42:08. She was the first female finisher in the 1982 Ironman Triathlon. Some of the marathoners Kinsey has coached are Scott Lyle (2:51:39), Pat Stewart (3:11:21), Ken O'Haure (3:20:38) and Cliff Griffin (3:26:42).

Kinsey's training plans:

Novice Marathoners
Sunday: Long run—16 to 20 miles
Monday: Rest
Tuesday: Track work
Wednesday: Easy run—6 miles
Thursday: Fast run—1 hour or more
Friday: Easy run—8 miles
Saturday: Rest

Experienced Marathoners
Sunday: Long run—16 to 20 miles
Monday: Rest
Tuesday: Track work
Wednesday: 8 miles
Thursday: 10 to 12 miles—hills, fartlek or cruise training. (Fartlek is a combination of fast and slow running, often done in the woods, and cruise training is steady running near race pace.)
Friday: 8 miles
Saturday: Rest, or 6 to 8 miles, easy

Elite Marathoners

Sunday: Long run—16 to 20 miles
Monday: Easy road run—8 miles
Tuesday (A.M.): 4 miles; **(P.M.):** Track work
Wednesday (A.M.): 4 to 6 miles; **(P.M.):** 8 miles
Thursday: 12 miles (hills, fartlek, cruise training)
Friday (A.M.): 4 to 6 miles; **(P.M.):** 8 miles
Saturday: Easy run—8 miles

Tip: A marathon is a long race. Get through 20 miles as comfortably as possible and then worry about the last 6 miles.

Diane Palmason
Englewood, Colorado

Diane Palmason coaches adult runners in the Denver area through her company Running Unlimited. Previously, she was director of the Canadian Association for Advancement of Women in Sport for Sport Canada. Palmason ran on the Canadian national team at the Commonwealth Games in 1954, when the longest distance event for women was 220 yards. Twenty-two years later, she switched to distance running and set Canadian masters records at distances from 800 meters to 80 kilometers, including a marathon best at age 46 of 2:46:23. Marathoners she has coached include Katie Kilbane (3:13:35) and Debbie Kallase (3:31:46).

Palmason's training plans:

Novice Marathoners

Sunday: Long run for 3-plus hours (including 5-10 minute walking breaks)
Monday: Recovery run—20 to 30 minutes
Tuesday: Medium run—45 to 60 minutes
Wednesday: Recovery run—20 to 30 minutes; plus strength training
Thursday: 4 to 9 miles at marathon pace
Friday: Deepwater pool running—40 minutes
Saturday: Strength training

Experienced Marathoners

Sunday: Long run—18 to 22 miles (every other week)

Monday: Recovery run—5 to 7 miles
Tuesday: Interval training—4 × 2000 meters; 400 walk or jog between
Wednesday: Easy run—5 to 7 miles; circuit strength training
Thursday: Tempo run—4 to 6 miles (fast in the middle)
Friday: Deepwater pool running—50 minutes including 3 × 3:00 hard; 3:00 between (use a flotation device or tread water)
Saturday: 4 to 11 miles at marathon pace

Elite Marathoners

Sunday (A.M.): Long run—22 plus miles (every other week); **(P.M.):** Short recovery run—2 to 4 miles
Monday: Easy run—8 to 12 miles
Tuesday (A.M.): Easy run—3 to 4 miles; **(P.M.):** Interval training—5 × 2000; 400 walk or jog between
Wednesday (A.M.): Easy run—3 to 4 miles; **(P.M.):** Steady run—5 to 7 miles; circuit strength training
Thursday (A.M.): Easy run—3 to 4 miles; **(P.M.):** Tempo run—5 to 7 miles (fast in middle)
Friday: Deepwater pool running—60 minutes including 5 × 3:00; 3:00 between
Saturday: 5 to 12 miles at marathon pace

Tip: Combine flexibility and strength drills (skipping, bounding, high knees, etc.) with your running workouts.

Doug Renner
Westminster, Maryland

Doug Renner is the manager of the Pro Image in Westminster and also serves as head track and cross-country coach at Western Maryland College. While coaching at Westminster High School in 1985, his team won the girls' state track championships. One of his top runners is Steve Kartalia, who placed ninth in the 10,000 at the 1992 Olympic trials and made his marathon debut in the 1992 Twin Cities Marathon, placing tenth overall (2:23:08). Some of the marathoners Renner has coached are Mike Santoni (2:40:02) and Jenny Caple (3:05:22).

Renner's training plans:

Novice Marathoners
Sunday: Long run—8 to 10 miles

Monday: Easy run—3 to 5 miles, relaxed (warm up and cool down)
Tuesday: 4 × mile at 10-K pace; 2:00 rest between
Wednesday: 5 to 7 miles, relaxed
Thursday: 5 to 7 miles, relaxed
Friday: Hill repeats (see how many you can do in 20 minutes)
Saturday: 3 to 5 miles, relaxed

Experienced Marathoners
Sunday: Long run—10 to 12 miles
Monday: 5 to 7 miles, relaxed (warm up and cool down)
Tuesday: 4 × mile at 10-K pace; 1:00 rest between
Wednesday: 5 to 7 miles, relaxed
Thursday: 5 to 7 miles, relaxed
Friday: Hill repeats (see how many you can do in 30 minutes)
Saturday: 3 to 5 miles, relaxed

Elite Marathoners
Sunday: Long run—12 to 15 miles
Monday: 5 to 7 miles relaxed (warm up and cool down)
Tuesday: 5 × mile at 10-K pace; 1:00 rest between
Wednesday: 5 to 7 miles, relaxed
Thursday: 8 to 10 miles, relaxed
Friday: Hill repeats (see how many you can do in 30 minutes)
Saturday: 5 to 7 miles, relaxed

Tip: Focus on keeping your running form as smooth and consistent as possible.

Patrick Joseph Savage
Oak Park, Illinois

Pat Savage teaches at Niles West High School in suburban Chicago and also coaches cross-country there and at nearby Oakton Community College. He is a member of the Illinois cross-country and track coach's Hall of Fame and has coached 23 National Junior College Athletic Association All-Americans. He also trains the Niles West/Oakton Runners Club. Marathoners Savage has coached include: Jukka Kallio (2:27:37), Tomasz Gnabel (2:31:28), Steve Rosenblum (2:34:15), Valerie Golbus (2:51:41) and Lise Monat (2:58:23).

Savage's training plans:

Novice Marathoners
Sunday: 18 to 22 miles
Monday: 30 to 45 minutes, fartlek
Tuesday: 30 to 45 minutes, easy
Wednesday: 30 to 45 minutes, including hills
Thursday: 30 to 45 minutes, easy
Friday: 30 to 45 minutes, easy
Saturday: Rest

Experienced Marathoners
Sunday: 18 to 22 miles
Monday: 6 × 1000 meters, 3:00 jog between
Tuesday: 45 minutes, easy
Wednesday: 45 minutes, fartlek
Thursday: 45 minutes, easy
Friday: 30 to 45 minutes, tempo run
Saturday: Rest

Elite Marathoners
Sunday: Long run—18 to 22 miles
Monday: 8 × 1000; 3:00 jog between
Tuesday: 1 hour easy
Wednesday: 75 minutes fartlek
Thursday: 1 hour, easy
Friday: 75 minutes, tempo run
Saturday: Rest or easy day

Tip: Shorter races build speed and act as tempo runs. A runner has to learn how to race.

Laszlo Tabori
Culver City, California

Laszlo Tabori was one of the world's top distance runners in the 1950s, competing for his native Hungary. In 1955, Tabori set a world record for 1500 meters with 3:40.8 and also ran a leg on the Hungarian 4 × 1500-meter relay team that broke the world record three times. At the 1956 Olympics, he placed fourth in the 1500 meters and sixth in the 5000, and then defected to the

United States with his coach Mihaly Igloi. Tabori now continues Igloi's coaching tradition with the San Fernando Valley Track Club. His athletes include Dave Barbiracki (2:16:20), Jacqueline Hansen (2:38:13) and Miki Gorman (2:39:11).

Tabori's training plans:

Novice Marathoners
Sunday: 1½-hour run
Monday: Intervals (150 to 300 meters, 50 to 100 meters rest between)
Tuesday: 30 minutes warm-up; 3 × 5:00 hard, 5:00 easy
Wednesday: 1 hour easy run
Thursday: Intervals (same as Monday)
Friday: 30 minutes easy run; 30 minutes fartlek
Saturday: Rest

Experienced Marathoners
Sunday: Long run—12 to 15 miles
Monday: 30 minutes easy run; 30 minutes fartlek
Tuesday: Intervals (200 to 400 meters; 100 to 200 meters rest between)
Wednesday: 45 minutes easy run
Thursday: Intervals (same as Tuesday)
Friday: 30 minutes easy run; 30 minutes fartlek
Saturday: 1½-hour easy run; 2 × 10:00 hard, 5:00 easy

Elite Marathoners
Sunday: Long run—15 to 18 miles
Monday: 20 minutes easy run; 40 minutes fartlek
Tuesday: Intervals (500 to 600 meters; 100 to 200 meters rest between)
Wednesday: 1:20 easy run
Thursday: Intervals (same as Tuesday)
Friday: Rest
Saturday: 30 minutes easy run; 4 × 5:00 hard, 5:00 easy

Tip: To avoid injuries, make sure that you warm up. Take your time doing it and be sure to stretch.

Robert H. Vaughan
Dallas, Texas

Bob Vaughan is an exercise physiologist at the Tom Landry Sports Medicine and Research Center. During the 1960s, he ran on a mile relay team that was ranked first in the nation his junior year, and second his senior year at Hillcrest High School in Dallas. He also ran the 440 (48.0) and 880 (1:53.7) at Texas A&M University. Some of the marathoners Vaughan has coached are Francie Larrieu Smith (2:27:35), Glenys Molly Quick (2:31:44), Sue Jackson (2:37:38) and Mary Knisely (2:37:58).

Vaughan's training plans:

Novice Marathoners
Sunday: 45 minutes to 1 hour
Monday: 1:15, easy
Tuesday: 45 minutes, easy
Wednesday: 1:30 to 1:45, easy
Thursday: 45 minutes, easy
Friday: Rest
Saturday: 2 to 3 hours

Experienced Marathoners
Sunday: 45 minutes, easy
Monday: 1:15, fartlek
Tuesday: 45 minutes, easy
Wednesday: 1:30, easy
Thursday: 1 hour, easy
Friday: 30 minutes, easy
Saturday: 2 hours or more

Elite Marathoners
Sunday: 1 hour, easy
Monday: 1:30, fartlek
Tuesday: 1 hour, easy
Wednesday: 45 minutes, easy
Thursday: 1:30 best aerobic effort
Friday: 30 to 40 minutes, easy
Saturday: 2 hours or more

Tip: Stay in good shape, pace yourself and drink, drink, drink.

CHAPTER 18

All-Time
FAVORITE
MARATHONS

O nce you've decided to train for a marathon, which one should you shoot for? Aside from the distance—which is 26 miles and 385 yards no matter what marathon you enter—races differ greatly. They can be flat or hilly, huge or small. They can take place in hot or cold weather or on a boring or beautiful course. And there's that indefinable quality: ambiance. Is there something that makes Boston more fun to run than New York? Or Athens? Or Honolulu?

The appeal of one race over another is tough to define, but when I sent questionnaires to the more than 50 coaches who provided information for this book, I asked them to try. I asked that they pick their ten all-time favorite marathons in the United States (as well as their ten favorites anywhere in the world). Here are their choices.

U.S. Races to Train For

1. Boston Marathon. No wonder that this April race hits the top of the list—it's *the* granddaddy of marathons. Started in 1897, Boston will celebrate its 100th anniversary in 1996. A point-to-point race from suburban Hopkinton to downtown Boston, the race course drops, levels off, climbs, drops again and generally beats runners to death. But we love it. Runners must meet strict standards to qualify. Contact: B.A.A. Boston Marathon, P.O. Box 1993, Hopkinton, MA 01748.

2. New York City Marathon. Founded by Fred Lebow in 1971 with a course that looped through Central Park, this November race expanded in 1976 to encompass all five boroughs: Staten Island through Brooklyn, the Bronx, Queens and into Manhattan. This is America's biggest distance event, with a field limited to 25,000 starters, many from foreign countries. Contact: New York Road Runners Club, P.O. Box 1388, GPO, New York, NY 10116.

3. Chicago Marathon. This flat and fast course is popular with runners and produced several world records in the mid-1980s. Budget cutbacks now prevent Chicago from attracting as many run-for-pay athletes; nevertheless, the marathon has grown in stature because of a caring attitude. Chicago's lakefront provides a splendid backdrop for this autumn race. Contact: Chicago Marathon, c/o Carey Pinkowski, 214 West Erie, Chicago, IL 60610.

4. Los Angeles Marathon. For years, Los Angeles hosted several small marathons but no big events. The 1984 Olympics prompted the city to go big league two years later, establishing a race that begins and ends at the Los Angeles Coliseum, passing through Hollywood. This race, run in early March, is America's second-biggest marathon, with 20,000 starters, any one of whom may be a soap opera star. Contact: Los Angeles Marathon, 11110 West Ohio Avenue, Suite 100, Los Angeles, CA 90025.

5. Twin Cities Marathon. This October race starts in Minneapolis and finishes in St. Paul, following a twisting course past lakes and along the Mississippi River. Autumn leaves are in full color, allowing race promoters to bill the race as "the most beautiful urban marathon in the country." Extra prize money for masters attracts the over-40 set. Contact: Twin Cities Marathon, 708 North 1st Street, Suite 238, Minneapolis, MN 55401.

6. Columbus Marathon. Site of the 1992 men's Olympic Trials, Columbus, Ohio, has a course that goes out and back on three different loops, passing the start/finish at 13 and 23 miles. Cool autumn weather and a flat course generally guarantee fast times. Contact: Columbus Marathon, c/o Joan Riegel, P.O. Box 26806, Columbus, OH 43226.

7. (tie) Grandma's Marathon. Midwest runners like Grandma's because its late June date allows more training time than other spring races. The point-to-point course follows the north shore of Lake Superior and ends in downtown Duluth near Grandma's Saloon & Deli, from which the race gets its name. Contact: Grandma's Marathon, P.O. Box 16234, Duluth, MN 55816.

7. (tie) Marine Corps Marathon. You'll go home loving the Marine Corps after this November race. The Corps provides the politest, snappiest, friendliest volunteers who ever offered a runner a cup of water. The course starts and finishes near the Iwo Jima Monument in Arlington, Virginia, and passes most of Washington's sights worth seeing. Contact: Marine Corps Marathon, P.O. Box 188, Quantico, VA 22134.

9. Houston-Tenneco Marathon. Site of the 1992 women's Olympic Trials, Houston offers a flat and pleasant loop course that wanders away from and back to the downtown area. The weather in this Gulf town can be unpredictable in late January— cool and windy one year, hot and humid the next—but it sure beats winter running up north. Contact: Houston-Tenneco Marathon, P.O. Box 2511, Houston, TX 77252.

10. (tie) Honolulu Marathon. Every runner's dream destination, Honolulu is particularly hospitable to first-time finishers and those finishing slow, often keeping the finish clock running eight hours or more. Despite a 5:30 A.M. start in December, the race is hot, humid and sunny, but everyone expects it and doesn't let the weather bother them. Go to enjoy the aloha spirit, and run your PR elsewhere. Contact: Honolulu Marathon Association, 3435 Waialae Avenue, #208, Honolulu, HI 96816.

10. (tie) Pittsburgh Marathon. A challenging (that means hilly) course, this early May race remains within city limits, crossing three bridges and roaming through Polish and Russian neighborhoods en route to a finish in Point State Park where the Monongahela, Allegheny and Ohio rivers meet. This is a midsize race (2,771 starters in 1992) that's been getting bigger. Contact: Pittsburgh Marathon, c/o Leonard Duncan, 1001 Law & Finance Building, 4th Avenue, Pittsburgh, PA 15219.

The Ten Best Marathons Worldwide

When coaches were asked to rank their ten favorite marathons anywhere in the world, many races from the United States list also made it onto the second list. Here's what our coaches voted as the ten best marathons in the world.

1. Boston Marathon
   The Olympic Games marathon (tie)
3. New York City Marathon
4. World Championships
5. Chicago Marathon
6. Columbus Marathon
7. Berlin Marathon, Germany
   Fukuoka Marathon, Japan (tie)
9. Los Angeles Marathon
   Marine Corps Marathon (tie)

Obviously, only a talented few gain entry to the Olympics or World Championships, and the Fukuoka marathon is limited to a few hundred very fast men (no women). For information on the Berlin Marathon, usually held in September, you can contact Marathon Tours, 108 Main Street, Charlestown, MA 02129.

Choosing Your Marathon

You may or may not want to aim for one of these all-time favorite marathons. You may prefer to pick a race that's close to home or one some of your friends are going to be running.

Although many marathons are open to anyone, this isn't true of all of them. To qualify for Boston, for example, you have to meet time standards, and New York uses a lottery to select its field of 25,000. Some other races limit the number of starters and accept entries on a first-come, first-served basis.

Other than that, you can pick and choose from hundreds of races throughout the United States and the world. Every January *Runner's World* magazine runs a listing of the marathons for the upcoming year with dates and contact phone numbers and addresses. Whatever race you hope to enter, you should contact race organizers early, enclosing a self-addressed, stamped business-size envelope with your inquiry.

Enjoy your marathon!

SUNBURST

Fog. That's all I could see when I gazed out the window of the Holiday Inn in South Bend, Indiana, at 5:00 in the morning. It looked like we were inside a cloud. As we rode to the start of the Sunburst Marathon in the hotel van, one of the other runners said the temperature was 58°.

But every cloud has its ugly lining.

A few minutes before the marathon's start on the campus of Notre Dame University, within sight of the football field where Knute Rockne's legions played, only a short distance from the Golden Dome, I knelt on a gravestone in the cemetery near the starting line to retie my shoes.

The ritual shoe-tying—or rather *retying*—is one of my final acts before going to the line. I tie the laces of my racing shoes first when I don them ten minutes before the race. I jog some and do a few quick sprints, which loosens the laces. Then I tighten the laces and tie them again with a double knot—a square knot over the double knot. Methodical as always, I don't want to risk having my laces come untied in the middle of a marathon.

I removed the T-shirt I had worn to the line for warmth on the still-cool morning and set it down on the gravestone. It was one of my favorite shirts: gray with red-and-blue lettering announcing the Asbury Park 10-K, a race in New Jersey just up the beach from the home of running guru George Sheehan, M.D. I planned to return to the cemetery after the race to reclaim it (but of course, forgot).

I wore red shorts and a plain white singlet, no message front or back. I had also brought my floppy hat for protection against the sun. With the fog still offering protection, the hat seemed superfluous. Nevertheless, I tucked it into the back of my shorts, uncertain what another hour—or two or three hours—on the road might bring.

The Sunburst Marathon is kingpin for a number of events: a 5-K run, a 5-K walk, a 10-K run, a triathlon. Joyce Fox is the race director. Sunburst is sponsored by the *South Bend Tribune,* for which I write a weekly running column. All events combined attract more than 3,300 participants, but there were only 378 in the marathon itself. That's a comfortable size if you hope to run fast, because you can get to the starting line a few minutes before the start and not have to worry about being delayed by a huge pack before you cross the line. The downside to Sunburst is that it's run in June, in usually hot and humid weather that's not conducive to good times. But it seemed as though we might be lucky this day.

Ron Gunn, my marathon class teaching partner, was giving some final instructions, but I wasn't listening. Several members of the class were there on the line, but I hardly saw them. Usually at the start of any race, I'm in my own fog.

The gun sounded, or at least I suppose it did, because we began running along a tree-shaded road that looped through the Notre Dame campus. The course returns to the start after two miles, then aims for the St. Joseph River that winds through South Bend (which is so named because of its location on the south bend of the river). The course heads downriver, then reverses upriver, then reverses downriver again before returning to campus.

Early in the first mile, I found myself running beside Don Hendricks, the cross-country coach from Mishawaka High School, which competes in the same conference as the high school team I coach. Normally I don't like to talk while racing, feeling it interferes with my concentration, but I found myself chattering with Hendricks about our teams.

At the first water station, I walked to drink, letting Hendricks slip ahead of me. Swallowing a full cup of water, I checked my watch and calculated I had lost precisely seven seconds. I caught Hendricks halfway to the next water station and pulled ahead. He passed me again as I walked once more to drink.

I remembered the words of marathon coach Bill Wenmark: "Nobody who passes you walking through a water station will ever beat you."

My first miles had felt labored, but now I found a comfortable groove. Hendricks and I swapped places once more at the next water station about ten miles into the race, and he said as I passed: "You probably won't see me again."

I didn't know about that: The marathon has a way of punishing intemperate early behavior. Coming down a short hill toward the bank of the river several miles further, I turned left upstream and suddenly I was struggling.

My wife, Rose, stood beside the course at mile 13, with a can of Coke for me as planned. "I'm dying," I told her, "but don't worry. I'll finish."

It had turned ugly. The fog had burned away, and Sunburst was living up to its name. I reached for my cap, thankful I had not discarded it. I allowed my pace to slide. I had been punching the button on my digital watch dutifully every mile to record my pace for reference afterward, but I deliberately didn't look to see how fast I was running. I didn't want to find out on a day that was getting warmer by the minute.

I adopted a strategy I had found useful in other warm marathons. At each mile marker, I shifted from running to walking to offer myself brief moments of recovery. (The secret of this is to never slow to a walk without picking the precise point—a pole, a tree, a sign—when you will begin running again.) I got through the final half dozen miles of the Chicago Marathon the previous fall doing this at a near 8:00 pace.

Don Hendricks caught me. "I thought you weren't going to see me again," I shouted after his shadow as he pulled away from me.

But if you have flexible goals, you can never be disappointed. By now I had shifted my strategy from running a fast time and placing well to merely finishing. I began to focus on scenery continuing upriver into Mishawaka, the town bordering South Bend. Usually I pay little attention to scenery, but now I was struck by the beauty of the Sunburst course. Just before the turnaround, I looked out on the river. Two men were fishing, oblivious to us runners struggling nearby. I tried to visualize myself in their boat, which seemed to be operating in a cooler dimension than ours. The temperature was climbing, and there were no more clouds in the sky.

Rose appeared with another can of Coke. I tried to assure her that I was suffering no major problems—other than running slowly.

Somewhere around 20 miles, things clicked into place again. Strange, since this was the point where I was supposed to hit the Wall, but somehow I felt invigorated. Another runner whom I judged to be in my age group passed, then another. I decided to focus on these two old-timers and see if I could beat them to the line.

Soon they fell behind me. I was into marathon mind games. I began focusing on Don Hendricks, somewhere out of sight ahead. If I could catch him, I decided it would mean that my team would defeat his during the next cross-country season. Far ahead, I spotted a runner in blue shorts who looked like Hendricks. I pressed to catch him only to discover several miles later that it was a case of mistaken identity. I shifted my focus on another runner ahead.

When you're running well in a marathon, the mile markers appear unexpectedly. When things go badly, you have to chase them. You tell yourself, "I must have missed it." Then you spot the next marker and know you were wrong.

The mile markers had appeared easily during the first half of the race; I had been chasing them since then. But now I was in fast forward. I spotted the 23-mile marker and thought, "Already?" I saw 24 and was amazed: "So soon?" I began to think that I would run out of course before catching Hendricks.

Turning a corner toward the stadium, I spotted Mary Connolly cheering for me and other finishers. She is the runner who had praised my article on marathon recovery, whom I mentioned in the introduction. "Mary," I shouted. "I mention your name in the introduction to my next book." She seemed puzzled by my comment, but by now she understands.

I had already begun to look beyond the finish line. Frank Shorter has said, "You're not ready to think about your next marathon until you've forgotten your last one." That already had begun to happen. Approaching Notre Dame stadium in the final mile, I began to wonder what that next marathon would be? Twin Cities? Chicago? Honolulu?

The Sunburst Marathon finishes on the football field on emerald grass. Fewer fans were in the stands than there would be on a football weekend, but I raised one arm as a victory sign crossing the finish line anyway. Somehow it did not disappoint me that my time was maybe a half hour slower than I might have anticipated in cool weather, on a downhill course, with the wind at my back. I was still in a marathoner's high as I grabbed for a soft drink, a banana, cookies and yogurt, before sitting down to untie my shoes. There was blood staining the front of one of them. I discovered my feet covered with blisters, caused undoubtedly by the heat. Strange, I had felt no pain while running.

Returning to the hotel, I called Don Hendricks to confirm that he, indeed, had finished before me. His time was seven minutes faster. "I don't care," I told him. "Our team is still going to beat yours next fall."

As I hung up the phone, I couldn't wait to run my next marathon.

It had been a good day for a run.

ABOUT THE AUTHOR

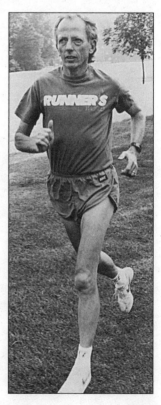

Hal Higdon, senior writer for *Runner's World* magazine, went out for his high school track team in 1947 and never stopped running. He won Midwest Conference championships while at Carleton College and has continued to win national and world titles, including running a 2:29 marathon at age 49 to win his age group at the 1981 World Veterans Championships in New Zealand. He was the first American to finish the Boston Marathon in 1964, placing fifth. He has run more than a hundred marathons (but doesn't remember the *exact* number).

Higdon is also a prolific writer, having published more than two dozen books on subjects as diverse as Civil War history and management consulting. His most recent books on running include *Run Fast* and *The Masters Running Guide*. In addition to writing frequently for *Runner's World,* Higdon also writes articles for *Snow Country, Boys' Life, American Health* and *Travel & Leisure.*

He lives with his wife, Rose, in Michigan City, Indiana, and writes a running column for an area newspaper, the *South Bend Tribune.*

INDEX

Note: Page references in **boldface** indicate tables.